The Extra Mile

The Journals of H.J.G. Geggie, M.D.
Medicine in Rural Quebec 1885–1965

Edited by Norma and Stuart Geggie
1987

Revised by Norma Geggie
2007

Copyright© 2007, Norma Geggie
Wakefield, Québec
Printed in Canada

ISBN 978-0-9693236-2-4

Canadian Cataloguing in Publication Data
Geggie, H. J. G. (Harold James Gugy), 1886–1966
    The Extra Mile : the Journals of H.J.G. Geggie, M.D. : Medicine in
Rural Quebec, 1885–1965 / edited by Norma and Stuart Geggie; revised
by Norma Geggie.

First edition published 1987, revised 2007.
ISBN 978-0-9693236-2-4

1. Geggie, H. J. G. (Harold James Gugy), 1886–1966. 2. Medicine,
Rural—Practice—Québec (Province). 3. Medicine, Rural—Québec
(Province)—History. 4. Physicians—Québec (Province)—Wakefield
Region—Biography. 5. Physicians (General practice)—Québec
(Province)—Biography. 6. Wakefield Region (Québec)—Biography.

I. Geggie, Norma II. Geggie, Stuart, 1925–1997. III. Title.

R464.G35A3 2007   610.92   C2007-903877-8

Published with financial assistance of the *Ministère de la culture et des
communications du Québec* and the *Gatineau Valley Historical Society*.

Table of Contents

GVHSIB 00844

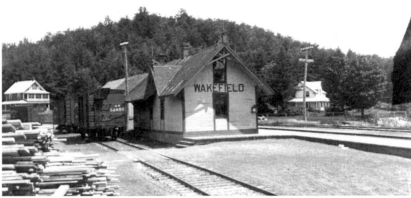

Wakefield Station in 1911.

Editor's Introduction

THE BABY, BORN OCTOBER 2, 1886, at Beauport, Quebec, was the second son of his parents, James Geggie and Leila Gugy. James had inherited from his Scottish father the ethic of hard work, scholarship, and a strict code of living, and was to pass these on to his children. He worked until his death as office manager for James Ross and Co., shipping magnates in Quebec. Leila Gugy was a leader, ahead of her times; proud of her forbears who had fought at Louisburg in 1758, at Quebec in 1759, at Chateauguay in 1812, and who later had contributed to their community in political and legal matters. With no male heir to continue the Gugy name, she gave it to each of her four children.

Into this background Harold James Gugy Geggie was born. Growing up and working on the family farm at Beauport, he was a reluctant student until his decision to study medicine at McGill brought a dogged determination to succeed. Upon graduation, with the gold medal in clinical medicine, he came to Wakefield to assist an ailing Dr. Hans Stevenson. He saw this as an opportunity to work with an experienced man and to grow into the profession of caring for the needy.

He was a shy young man, somewhat lacking in confidence. On the untimely death of the man he saw as his "Preceptor" and his tutor, he thought himself trapped. Doubted by some for his youthfulness, resented by others for trying to fill the Old Doctor's boots, he remained determined to help his people under often impossible conditions, alone and overworked. He was to become a legend in his own time, loved in turn by his people. He lived to see the fulfilment of his dream of a hospital, supported by and supporting his community, and to see his three sons and a grandson follow him in his choice of profession. Into his notebooks he poured out his heartbreaks, his frustrations, his accomplishments and his compassion for the people.

The original tales, penned in 1960 and published a quarter of a century later, hold a strong interest today, close to fifty years after they were written. The poignant stories, read and reread, and recently told in a one-man theatrical presentation, inform us of the desperate struggle to cope with conditions in health care one hundred years ago. They stress the changes in society and in our medical system and serve as an inspiration.

Norma Geggie, 2007

Dear Christ, who reign'st above the flood
Of human tears and human blood,
A weary road these men have trod,
O house them in the home of God.

— from Requiescant by Canon Frederick George Scott
    In a field near Ypres
    April 1915

Author's Preface and Dedication

THIS BOOK HAS BEEN A-WRITING for more than fifty years. It has been my companion throughout my years of medical practice: while I drove horses under the stars on cold winter nights; on drowsy hot summer afternoons; threading a way along soft, almost bottomless spring roads; mired up to the axles—waiting for the slow arrival of the team of horses to pull me out; or bumping over iron-hard ruts of frozen November roads, hoping the ever-to-be-suspected crown gear would hold out 'til my journey's end. At all hours, on the roads or at bedsides, dozing curled up on the kitchen floor on my sleigh rugs, sitting up in the middle of the night, with head resting on the steering wheel, or half waking, half sleeping, lying on the soft grassy roadside; over all the years this book has been writing itself. Much of it has been written in episodes. Much of it has been written and rewritten with changes and additions, but with little or no invention; and much has been carried only in thought, triggered by the daily doings. Sometimes one can't help writing a book—it writes itself.

There is a greater reason for writing a book on rural medical practice. There have been so many changes over the past fifty years; economic and social, professional and scientific. Two world wars, economic inflations following them, followed in turn by depressions, one enormous and worldwide, and one seriously threatening; all have changed humanity's outlook, reaching into even the remote rural parts. What went into the making of a doctor before the turn of the 20th century, or in its first decade, or its fourth or fifth decades? These things deserve to be recorded.

Can I portray my Preceptor, Dr. Hans Stevenson, the Old Doctor who died so young of overwork, while his brothers and sisters all lived to over eighty, several into their nineties and one to over a century? Can I portray my mother and my father, whose way of life gave me my strongest beliefs and prejudices? Can I do justice

5

to the sacrifices, the devotion, the trust of those whose lives touched mine so closely, those whose stories, in part, will need to be told? Should I let the story remain with me, destroy what is already written, let it follow the rest to the inevitable end and never let it see the light of day? Yet might not the written record be of some use, if only to one reader, some grandchild over the long future? Might it not be of some use to one curious reader wanting to know how people lived at the turn of the 20th century, before the wars, before the wide use of electricity, oil, internal combustion engines; before aviation, broadcasting, before X-rays, the sulfas, vitamins and antibiotics? Was medicine—rural medicine—possible at all before these things? Perhaps it is worth writing down.

In all this, my thanks and gratitude are due to my wife who made our necessary way of life possible; who, just as her mother and her aunt Mary did before her, has spent her life making her man's life easier. How many times when her father or I happened to be out on the road, have these three, one or other, watched the wood fires, had the house comfortable and a meal ready when we reached home? How many times had they a fresh team ready for us to start out again? Their devotion to our patients, through us, has been life-long. This book then, is dedicated to my wife, Ella Stevenson, to her mother, Margaret Cann Stevenson, to her aunt, Mary Stevenson Shouldice, who, one after the other since 1880, have done so much to make rural medicine possible in this Gatineau valley. There was of course, another woman, my mother Leila Gugy Geggie.

Harold J.G. Geggie MD, 1960

The Promise

"FOLLOW THE THREE TELEPHONE wires for about ten miles; turn right and follow the two wires another ten; follow the remaining wire past the church to its end. Two miles further on, turn right up a steep, rocky, winding hill. Baptiste lives in the second white-washed log house at the end of the road." So directed my Preceptor, and with seventy five dollars' worth of anti-diphtheritic serum at my feet, four days after graduation, I started out on my first big solo assignment. I had not yet gone more than the first few miles along this road; all was new to me, new people, new farms, new mountains and lakes and streams. If the country was new, so was I, or I was made to feel very new indeed by the interest aroused in the people rocking on their front verandas, or playing horseshoes or croquet as I drove by with the Old Doctor's well-known team.

I could almost sense the thoughts going through the heads of old and young alike. "The new doctor. Too young; he'll never take the Old Doctor's place in these hills. He's not married; no good." It was a very self conscious, a very young doctor indeed who drove quickly by on that hot June Sunday afternoon long ago. As to the young man's thoughts: "Three wires, ten miles, right, two wires, ten miles, one wire, five miles past the church, crooked hill, three miles further, the last house on the road."

Did these corkscrew roads never end? Did they not just go on and on again? Around the hills, over the hilltops to avoid swamp and corduroy, around lakes, across rushing streams, on queer bridges showing signs of spring washouts. Here and there, glimpses between the crowding hills, the flat meadow lands, old beaver meadows perhaps, with an alder lined creek winding and twisting along to the bigger creeks and lakes below; creeks full of trout, no doubt, if one had a moment to try them. On and on, thinking of this and that; flowering weeds along the way, climbing wild grapes, flowering chokecherries and wild apples, tall pines left there perhaps because they had branched out widely and so did not make good logs; swamps thick with cedar and tamarack, croaking frogs, singing birds, a wild hare with his shining new summer coat, loping along with his long skinny legs. Then, in spite of all this came thoughts of the job in hand, to which all this newness was only incidental. Diphtheria? Diagnosis, quarantine laws, complications, early and late, sequelae, death rate.

Treatment was simple; enough serum at two dollars per thousand units, and needing twenty to forty thousand. Still, the problem was as yet far off, beyond the miles yet to cover. Time enough when I got to the boy. Three hours driving in the heat brought me to Long Lake, at the upper end of which stood the church, one of my landmarks; only five or six miles further to go. In less than an hour I must examine, diagnose and treat my first big case. I felt very small indeed, very inadequate. I found the famous unnamed hill. For miles around it was just The Hill. I started up its sandy, stony winding way. The tired horses were foam flecked, for I had pushed them hard in the heat. As they kept climbing I glanced behind at the valley below and noticed the dark storm clouds

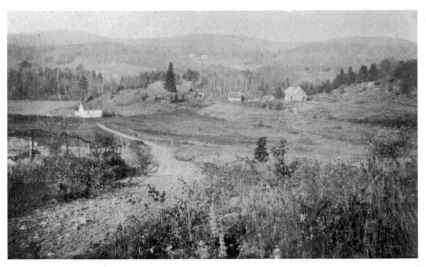

A typical Gatineau road, c.1911.

gathering to the northwest. Birds were quiet, sensing the storm; even the horses began to feel it coming and put on a little spurt when at last we reached the top of the hill. Perhaps they remembered the stable they'd been in just a week ago when Marie Ange had been ill. In preparation for their feed of oats, a handy water hole made a worthwhile stopping place while we all had a much-needed drink.

"Never neglect your horses," my Preceptor said in his quiet way as we drove one day. "Don't ask for food for yourself. You can always get along; the horses can't. All depends on them." I felt the horses thought the same of him. Buster always kept one ear turned backwards to hear his master's voice urging him on.

But my hour of trial was at hand. I drove into the sandy clearing on the lakeshore, where stood Baptiste's log house, white against the darkening western sky. Even as I looked, the sky was split by lightning, and low growling thunder made the collie dog scuttle for the barn to hide in the hay. Horses seen to, I made my way into the house with my heavy bag, in which I carried everything but the nurse and the patient, and my parcel of precious serum.

The house was one large room; the whole lower floor in one, about twenty by twenty-four feet and eight feet in height, with red painted beams across the ceiling, fresh, white-washed logs within and without. A steep stairway went up to the attic room. In one corner was a wide bed in which lay my patient, gasping and struggling for breath, a dusky, muddy pallor about his mouth, the wings of his nose going back and forth in his distress. I could see at a glance that I had an almost hopeless case. Unless the serum worked a real miracle this time, there was not much to do. Both tonsils and soft palate, and as far down the throat as was easily seen, were covered with the thick grey-green membrane, curling here and there at the edges to show the bloody bed beneath. The odour, the stink, typical and special, never-to-be-forgotten when once smelt, was diagnostic. The pulse racing, almost not to be counted, faltered now and then, and the breathing was laboured. "He only went to bed yesterday," said the mother. "Of course he had a cold in his head and his nose was running all week. It scalded all his lip, you see, but he was not real sick. He went down to the church to catechism on Thursday; walked down."

I was busy drawing huge doses of serum into my largest syringe. This given, I could look about me. The horses had to eat, so I had to wait. Besides, the far off storm was getting closer. Already the trees were beginning to complain in the gusts that came from any and every direction. Clouds came sailing over, piling and splitting to show an unearthly splendour of sunshine, blotted out the next moment when a greater, darker mass came up. Lightning split the sky, the ever nearer thunder rolled.

I had given the serum only half an hour earlier, and of course there was no response as yet. Something must be done. Swabbing the throat with ferric chloride suggested itself, easier than blowing Flowers of Sulphur down the throat, as used to be done in pre-serum days. Strychnine or camphor, to keep the heart going; desperate, useless steps all of them. Perhaps my helplessness showed in my face, not yet schooled into remaining expressionless before disaster, too young at the job.

An uncle standing by murmured, "J'irai chercher le Curé," and he went out into the gathering storm to harness his horse and cross the mountains eight miles to the next parish where the Curé had gone that Sunday for early Mass, and was staying over to hear confessions. He was not long gone when the storm burst over our heads. The lake water, seemingly flattened 'til then, all of a sudden jumped and rushed up the shore, making such a noise that my patient's struggles seemed stilled. Rain on the roof made a rattle I shall never forget; a pool of water gathered under one window, and a thin stream soon stretched across the room. The door, being on the lee side of the room, remained open, and through it I could watch the leaping waves, lit up ever and again by the flashes of lightning.

Quietly, and without emotion, the mother placed a chair in the centre of the room, and covered it with a white cloth. In the centre she placed a glass dish for Holy Water at the feet of a small statue of the Virgin in her blue cloak, holding the Holy Child on her left arm, her right arm by her side, beckoning as it were with her palm, "Come unto me." On either side a lighted Holy candle guttered and fluttered with the fitful draughts from the open door. Pouring Holy Water into the glass dish, she handed the bottle to her husband, who went out into the storm to sprinkle the four corners of the house, the windows, the chimney and the open doorway while she, taking a spray of dried evergreen saved from Palm Sunday, sprinkled the four corners of the room, the bed, and her boy, each doing his or her best to avert the rage of the storm.

Presently Baptiste came in, dripping wet, and joined his wife on his knees by the altar, beads in hand, repeating again, "Je vous salue Marie. Je crois en Dieu. Notre Père qui êtes aux cieux..." (Our Father who art in Heaven). In a few moments there was a pool of water dripping from his clothing onto the floor about them as they prayed. I was steaming the boy's throat by then. The coal oil lamp on the floor was boiling a pot hanging over it, the air, heavy with Tincture Benzoin made an incense for the fountain of prayer. By now the storm was rolling further away to the east across the lake. Little lulls began to be noticeable in the respirations of the boy. I had given all my serum, shot my best bolt as it were.

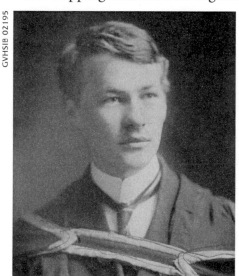

GVHSIB 02195

Harold Geggie at graduation, June 11, 1911.

Out of the storm came the uncle, dripping wet, with his wet hands wiping his face. He had seen Monsieur le Curé; he could not come. The boy was in a good way; he would die in peace without him. He would pray for him. Giving his message, wet as he was, he joined the kneeling parents and together they joined in the Litany for the Dying, the mother reading the priest's part, the men mumbling the answers. The storm was further away now, thunder still growling far across the lake, lightning still flashing on the other side of the water. It was nearly midnight, my boy unconscious. Nothing I could do, or even pretend to do, remained; I watched and waited. The breathing slowed and the pulse stumbled.

Down the stairs came Marie Ange, staggering with emotion, straining her diphtheria paralysed throat in a loud whisper. "I have killed him by bringing the disease home from town! I have killed him! I will give my life, if God wills it, to the care of the sick. Even if Amède has no health, I will marry him and look after him! That will be my penance." She bent over her dying brother, making her promise and repeating: "Je vous salue Marie. Je crois en Dieu. Notre Père qui êtes aux cieux…"

I went out across the wet sands in the dying storm, to the stable where the horses were contentedly munching in their well-filled manger. Throwing myself on the pile of hay I wept. My first case, a failure.

Marie Ange kept her promise, she married Amède. She is still keeping her promise after forty-five years, looking after the sick.

So began Dr. Harold James Gugy Geggie's half-century of medical practice in the Gatineau Valley. (Editor's note)

Family Roots

MY MOTHER LAY AWAITING my birth, while my father was out looking for the doctor. Years later, in a joking mood on my birthday, my father said that perhaps I should be celebrating the 3rd of October and not the 2nd, for he had first seen me after midnight, when he came in from his fruitless search. Mrs. McVeigh, the midwife, who had ushered me into the world, presented me to him. If, however, I was born on the 2nd October, 1886, a Saturday, as my mother insisted, perhaps I have lived up to the saying "Saturday's child works hard for a living". I was third in the family, the second boy, to be followed in 1888 by a sister, and yet another in 1891. Four of us lived to adulthood, but Annie, the youngest, died of burns when her clothes caught fire from a candle. I was slightly scorched trying to put out the fire. Thus I became acquainted with accidents and subsequent death, and the horror of burn accidents remained with me.

Beauport, the village in which I was born, is about three miles down the St. Lawrence River from Quebec. It was first settled in 1634 by Robert Giffard, a doctor, who had come to Quebec some years before and had liked the duck hunting along the tidal beaches of the St. Lawrence. He was the first seigneur in Canada, and built a small house on the banks of the Rivière des Ours. Returning to France, he secured the grant of the seigneury from the French king, and brought back a party of colonists to fulfil his seigneurial responsibility. In 1634, he began his Manor House, putting into the corner stone a lead plate which was subsequently found in the fire of 1879, and is now in the National Archives in Ottawa.

My mother, Leila Gugy, was born in this manor house in 1854. She was brought up with a deep interest in history, in genealogy, in medicine and the land. The first member of the Gugy family to arrive in Canada was Conrad Gugy, a Swiss German soldier who was present at the sieges of Louisbourg and Quebec. Liking Canada, he bought seigneuries near Three Rivers and settled down to spend the rest of his days. He never married, and his brother Bartholomaeus, a Swiss Guard to King Louis XVI, came after the French Revolution, with his wife and son Louis, to take over the property.

Louis Gugy served as Sheriff of Three Rivers, and later of Montreal, and he and his son took part in de Salaberry's victory over the Americans in the War of 1812 at Chateauguay. This son, B.C.A. Gugy, born in Yamachiche in 1796, was my grandfather, a Montreal and later a Quebec lawyer, and a militia Major in the Revolution of 1837. He was completely bilingual, and sympathetic to the French Canadian aspirations. Although despising their Roman Catholicism, my grandfather married, in turn, a French Roman Catholic, Sophie Louise Duchesnay, and after her death, an Irish Roman Catholic, Mary McGrath (often spelt and pronounced "McGraw")—my grandmother.

I remember "Mémère" (we also had a Scottish "Grandmama" in Ottawa), and we were a bilingual family. I remember Mémère sitting up in bed at night by candlelight, gasping for breath with asthma, smoking stramonium leaves in a clay pipe. I remember the struggle for breath gradually getting easier as the drug began to take effect. She died in the early 1890s, probably my earliest contact with the facts of old age, illness, and death in my young experience. She was born in Prince Edward Island shortly after her parents emigrated from Ireland. She never learned to speak much French, although she lived in French-speaking Canada for all her married life.

In religion, although an Anglican, my mother was most tolerant of all beliefs, though not always of religious organizations; for example, Roman Catholic Orders and evangelistic societies. My paternal grandfather, Robert Currie Geggie, was a Reformed Presbyterian (Covenanter) who had come to Quebec from the lowlands of Scotland to teach school in 1832. On Saturdays he would walk to Valcartier, Stoneham, or Lake Beauport, to preach long sermons to the settlers the next day.

My father, James Geggie, one of eight children, had left school and become one of the earliest telegraph operators in Quebec. At the age of seventeen he joined Ross and Company, a shipping and general commercial firm in Quebec, where he remained at a low salary for almost sixty years, until his death in 1915. Although born in Canada, he was very much a Scotsman, a silent man, a promiscuous steady reader. Although running the shipping business all week, he helped my mother run the farm, and her sister, my aunt, to run her adjoining farm, as well as a large limestone quarry to pave streets in Quebec city.

After dark in the evenings while we were at our lessons, my father would be close at hand reading the *Edinburgh Scotsman, The Guardian, The Spectator, The Montreal Witness*. Often some history lesson would bring up a point. It was rare when he could not fill in for us what the history books had left out: Garibaldi, McMahon, especially Lincoln, the Pretender; he made them all live for us. Lessons over, almost each night, my father would take down The Book, and in the voice kept by his generation especially for the occasion, we would hear the Old Testament stories: Saul and David, Ruth and Naomi, Abraham and Isaac, and the rest.

As I grew up we attended the Quebec Anglican Cathedral or St. Andrew's Presbyterian Church, alternately, with either or both parents. We did not get to church every Sunday, nor did we ever get to Sunday School. Nevertheless, each Sunday we had morning and evening prayers on our knees, with hymn singing and reading of the lessons, until we were perfectly familiar with most of the Anglican prayer book, and the hymns in common use at the time. These have remained as familiar as ever over the years; a background from which to think, often companions to pass the time while driving at night under the stars in winter, or to help keep awake on hot rainy nights in summer: *Lead Kindly Light, The Lord is My Shepherd, Work for the Night is Coming, Now Lettest Thou Thy Servant Depart in Peace, Unto the Hills Around,* and even *Rescue the Perishing,* although it seems a bit melodramatic.

Sunday was a queer, irrational mixture of Scottish narrowness and Anglican breadth. We played no games on Sunday inside or out, summer or winter. There were no card games, and no dancing, but in winter we took out our toboggans and sleighs, snowshoes and skates, much to the disgust of our aunt and uncle in Quebec, who expected us to be in the house on Sunday afternoon reading *Pilgrim's Progress* or some elevating sermons. In summer my parents took us, all five, to walk down across the farm to see the hay and grain growing, to note what was to be done the following day, and to see the calves, colts, sheep and poultry. Then, sitting under a tree "below the hill", my father would read to us *Lays of Ancient Rome, Lay of the Last Minstrel,* Tennyson's *The Brook, The Merchant of Venice, Midsummer Night's Dream,* and *Idylls of the King.* Long before going to school and reading these for myself, their music, if not the meaning, were part of me, old friends conjuring up my father's voice, conjuring up the shape of the hills, the trees and fields. They still do, after all these years.

Ours was not a "religious" house; we said no grace at meals; we were not given to attributing daily happenings to God's pleasure or displeasure. The responsibility was on us. If things went wrong, someone was to blame; if they went right, no less was expected of us. We got little praise if our school results were good, perhaps because none of us covered our brows with the leaves of scholarship in school. Geggies came second, never first. Public dances were taboo. Games took little time out of our lives. We were largely "stay-at-homes", but we shared a great measure of contentment.

The outstanding thing about my mother, in many ways so broad, so tolerant, so adaptable, was her absolute intolerance for alcohol and tobacco in any form. Gladly would she have seen both abolished from the earth by any effective measure. She was only more or less fair to the "trades". Apparently her lawyer father, B.C.A. Gugy, having seen the effects of alcohol upon family life, when his son was born put behind him all alcohol, even socially.

We grew up, as other children of the time, with a mixture of tolerances and prejudices, beliefs and misbeliefs, the results of which have been both good and bad. With more tolerance perhaps we would have done better, but I doubt that I would have grown up with the more or less crusading missionary spirit that brought me to my "corner of the woods" and kept me here the whole of my life.

A big influence on my life has been the consciousness of history and background. Our farm had been the seigneurial farm, and we were aware of its history. It had served as headquarters of General Montcalm in 1759, and was where he had spent his last night, while the first Gugy, with Wolfe, climbed Cape Diamond. The manor house was latterly the first insane asylum in Canada. It was rumoured that treasure had been hidden there, and the subsequent fire that destroyed the building, was attributed to treasure hunters. The house in which we lived was the birthplace of Colonel de Salaberry, Commander of the Canadian Militia at the battle of Chateauguay in the War of 1812, and under whom my grandfather had served as a very junior officer. We housed many historical mementoes: the plaque from the Giffard manor, the regimental flags of the militia regiment my grandfather commanded, a spike from the "Alert", an Arctic exploration vessel which had been burned on our Beauport beach, and some of Wolfe's cannon balls which had been turned up by our ploughs.

All these beginnings had their effect. In 1898–99 I was at high school on the Quebec Ramparts just outside the Citadel. The South African contingent was gathering in the Citadel, and as youngsters we used to spend the noon hour amongst the soldiers. We watched them sail from the King's Wharf, the whole thousand of them. Without doubt this background of history has affected my whole life and outlook, a background shaped by my parents and my surroundings.

My father was forty nine when I was born, and, in my eyes, an old man when I began to know him. His brown hair and square trimmed beard were already whitening, so that I always stood in awe of him, not fear; I always looked up to him, perhaps therefore, always tending to look up to those older or greater in experience than I. My father and I understood each other without the need for discussion. Only twice can I remember having a heart-to-heart talk with him. Once when about sixteen, I was in great trouble with geometry at school. He came to my room in the dark, where I was lying awake finding it impossible to face school the next day. He begged me to continue school, to make something more of myself than he was able to make of himself. Wisely, but much to my teacher's disgust, my parents agreed to my giving up geometry for the rest of the year. I have since been very sure that when the restless low period comes, as come it always does in a boy's or girl's life, some difficult decisions must be faced, something must give. It is luck if it is some minor issue like geometry.

Two weeks before my father died, when I was a doctor and nursing him after he had had a very serious attack of weakness from a gastric haemorrhage, he asked me, "What do the doctors say of me? Will I get better?" It was my father asking. I had been in practice only a few years: it was a hard question. Older consultants had held out no hope. What should I say? I could not lie. I told the truth. "Then I want to see your mother alone."

He had, over the past twenty years, been paying off a debt, money that he had forfeited on some promissory notes that he had endorsed for an office associate who had defaulted. My father's money had gone to educate the other man's sons. One thousand dollars remained to be paid and he was dying. He had kept silent over the years but he had to speak now. Bit by bit over the years, on a salary of twelve to fifteen hundred dollars a year, he had paid off many thousands. There have been many times when, as a doctor, I have got around the truth. I am thankful that for once I told the truth, and my father was able to relieve his mind of his heavy secret.

My mother was a good partner to my father, a complement to his Scottish austerity. Our communications were generally through my mother, an intermediary through whom decisions were made, but I always felt my father was thinking of me, guiding me; not a companion to me, one to look up to, to emulate. I had a good "team" behind me. At school as boys, my brother and I were undistinguished. When he was fifteen or sixteen my brother, of more robust build and character than I, kicked over the traces and would not stay in school. He entered a bank at eight dollars a month. I, who was more retiring and less assertive, hated the idea of going into business and meeting the public, and hated city life far from the land. As a lesser evil I kept on at school.

When I was seventeen and in my last year of school, most of the class were talking of going to college; I wasn't talking. The class was going to Montreal to play high school football. Somehow I went with the team to watch the game. Next day was a McGill sports day; we went to a song practice, saw McGill sports, and saw a thousand students. The ferment began to work; I too must go to McGill, but I must have a pass in geometry.

The day after I returned from Montreal I began working on my own: by Christmas I'd caught up with the class, and instead of losing that period, I was doing it. After Christmas a geometry test came up and as I put in my paper "Chubby" Young, my teacher, looking a fierceness I'm sure he did not feel, said "Geggie you've been studying Euclid; have the lesson ready for tomorrow." I answered with a very small "yes". In the June exam I got some 60% and was able to register that September at McGill for Arts and Medicine. Three years before this my brother had begun to work at his entry to study medicine at Laval. He was already in second year and went on to graduate in 1909. Why were we both interested in medicine?

Among my earliest recollections was a crowd of children and a few mothers around our kitchen table, with sleeves pushed up and my mother dabbing and scratching each arm with a drop of warm water and rubbing a dried scab of a previously successful vaccination in it. We all knew the story of Dr. Jenner, of Lady Wortley Montague, and of Napoleon's Italian army in 1796, which was successful against the smallpox-ridden Italian army because of vaccination. We knew of the smallpox epidemics in Quebec and Montreal in the 1880s. Any day we could see "Giroulx le picotté", or "Parent le picotté", neighbours whose faces were scarred by confluent smallpox.

A little later, one March day, our playmate was with us happy on the snowy hills. Less than a week later he was dead and buried: diphtheria. Diphtheria struck again ten days later in another friend; an expensive new French serum was made available by my mother who brought home the two empty vials. Two days later, as we passed the boy's home, he waved to us through the frosted window-pane. A cure had been effected by the serum.

Although I was bilingual, writing and spelling in French were not easy to someone who had learned the language phonetically. I got only 15% in my first year Arts French. Latin had been taken in stride in school; I had a good memory. In college, I just scraped through first year. I tried a supplemental in Latin five times without passing it, and took French and scientific German instead. I never got a B.A., but I did get enough of both Latin and German to add to my enjoyment of understanding French, German, and English.

In my last year at McGill I was fed up with hospital and city life; I wanted to get to work. I volunteered to the Grenfell Mission, at an isolated island base off the coast of Labrador, if I remember well. My training was not sufficient, and another got the job. Later I flirted with a mission in Honan under the Presbyterian Mission Board. Even after I was three years in practice, the Board canvassed me again, but I had found my "China" in Wakefield, and I refused the offer.

Often, looking back, have I decided that my whole path has been drifting, not choosing my way; never a decision this way or that, except in the problems for immediate action; a pawn in the scheme of things. Long ago, the form of address of the lower orders of monks to their superiors was, "Dear Father in God". My form of address to my Preceptor, Dr. Hans Stevenson could well have been "Dear father in medicine." I had seen Dr. Stevenson's appeal for assistance on the McGill noticeboard. Little thinking, I remarked to my roommate beside me, "There's a good job for someone, but I don't want it." Three weeks later I was in Wakefield looking for the job.

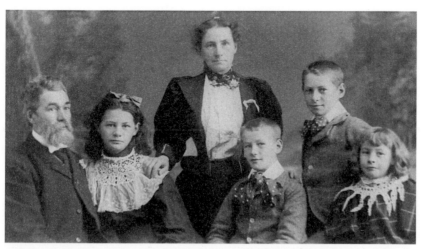

James and Leila Geggie with children, Lois, Harold, Conrad and Elsa. 1895.

Settlement

THE SMALL VILLAGE OF WAKEFIELD *nestles around the banks of the Gatineau River in the Province of Quebec, twenty miles north of Ottawa. Rising some one hundred miles further north, the Gatineau was late in being exploited for lumbering because of its many treacherous rapids and falls. The river winds its way south through rocky weathered hills, part of the Laurentian shield, and through enclosed fertile valleys to join the Ottawa River at Ottawa. It is to this day a beautiful river valley, and must have been magnificent when those first settlers made their way up it in the 1830s, with the fine stands of red and white pine extending along its course. The townships of Wakefield and Masham had been described in land applications as early as 1793, but it was not until some years after Philemon Wright and his associates had settled on the north bank of the Ottawa River in 1800, that a progression began in opening up land on either side of the river. Within thirty to forty years, despite the treacherous river and difficult terrain, small pockets of settlers had cleared land, built log cabins, and were beginning to develop communities at distances of five to ten miles apart. The farms were hidden from one another by the hills, and thus seemed isolated. People of like religious belief claimed land adjacent to each other, and settlements developed of people from Southern Ireland, Scotland, England and Northern Ireland, and French families moving up from Lower Canada. Each of these pockets of development was three or four miles from the next, and in each, the establishment of a church or meeting place had high priority and served a vital role in the lives of the people, both spiritually and socially. Most farms were of fifty to one hundred acres, with some of two hundred acres; but only about a quarter of the land would be cultivated. Each farmer had a horse or two, a few cattle and pigs and occasionally a few sheep. Roads, or the lack of them, compounded the problem of isolation, small streams had to be forded, and in some seasons would have been impassable. By the 1860s and 1870s, thriving villages had developed in such places as Masham, Wakefield, North Masham (Rupert) and Farrellton, with sawmills, grist mills and a variety of trades-people. Lumber merchants had extended their territory far north. There were many prosperous farms and good farmers, but as one moved back from the river, where the soil was thinly spread over the rocks and had been rapidly exhausted by cultivation, many subsistence farms were to be found. The large families had helped to clear the fields of stones, but crops were meagre; the prime timber had been cut, and the male members of the household needed to spend the winter months in northern lumber camps to supplement the income. At such times the women suffered greatly from isolation, loneliness and overwork, as they attempted to carry out the routine chores both inside and outside their homes, as well as caring for large families.*

These pioneers developed a tremendous self sufficiency, and a philosophy of acceptance of the problems and tragedies that befell them, partly because of their deep religious faith, and partly because of an upbringing in rigorous circumstances in their home countries. These were the people with whom Dr. Hans Stevenson had grown up, and this was the country where he chose to practice. Preceded by "Little" Dr. Stephen Wright in 1860, then by "Big" Dr. Falls, he returned to his country in 1885. This, too, was the country that Dr. Harold Geggie first saw in 1911, on his arrival, intending to assist the older doctor for two years, and staying, fifty-five. (**Editor**)

The Stevensons

AMONG THE TWENTY HOUSEHOLDERS, mostly from Ireland, who had settled in the township of Wakefield in the 1830s, were two brothers, Thomas and John Stevenson, from Killeleah, County Down, Ireland. They had settled on six hundred acres, lakes and mountains, fertile clay valleys and loamy hillsides covered by dense bush, pine trees and spruce, cedar swamps, maple trees and elm. The brothers were cutting trees on the river bank, when around the bend came two canoes, laden with the effects of a newly arrived immigrant family. In one canoe sat a young woman. Women were few and far between at the time. "There goes your wife, John," quipped Thomas.

The Pritchards, in the canoes, took over a large area four miles higher up the river, one of the most fertile valleys in our country. As it turned out, it was Thomas himself, not John, who married Ann Pritchard. There are family tales of Ann, who, fearful of the danger to Thomas from wolves, preferred to remain alone all night in their log cabin, rather than have him walk home in the bush after exchanging labour with neighbours two miles away. Ann became the local midwife, and would go off with a basket of food on her arm, to visit a newcomer or perhaps to nurse a sick neighbour.

Neighbours did come, Maxwells and McClintons, O'Connors and McGarrys, McKittricks, Clarkes and Milnes. Thomas became in time the local arbiter in disputes over fences and boundaries, the counsellor in family troubles and church elder. Ann told a story of Thomas coming home from a long day's ploughing in the autumn: "Ann, I've decided not to smoke any more; 'tis a filthy habit. I ploughed my pipe under in the furrow and I'll smoke no more!" There is also a story of Ann and Thomas setting out on horseback for Sacrament Sunday, twenty-five miles away at the County Seat, when horse paths were finally cut along our river.

They carried with them, in their saddle bags, some farm produce, and brought back on Monday morning a bag of salt, some tea, and some cloth.

Ann, as a grandmother, would gather the grandchildren in her own room at the farm, and read long chapters from The Book, the wee girls only holding out because they knew that at the end of the session there would be a hard peppermint candy to suck. Often at these sessions Thomas would come by and interject, "Let the children go now Ann, they've had enough!" But Ann would pay not the slightest attention, not so much as raising her eyes from the page, not until the chapter was through.

There is too, the tale of friendly Indian encampments in their orchard; the Indians were travelling up river to their trapping grounds near the headwaters, as they had done for hundreds of years before the white man came.

Probably the last link with Killeleah was in 1853, about the time Ann's youngest son was born. Thomas's brother, Hans, arrived from Ireland. The new baby was called Hans. Learning to read at the spinning wheel, often with a tallow dip (the "slut" it was called), he became in turn a school teacher and then a doctor. From 1880 to 1911 he supplied the country's needs for medical care, driving horses, at times a single in a two wheeled sulky, at times a team in an open buggy. Winter with heavy snow and cold winds was no hindrance to him. Where there was need, he was to be found, "beau temps, mauvais temps", for at least half the population spoke little English. He died, worn out, aged fifty-nine. One of his sisters passed the century, all his brothers and sisters passed four score, four of them passed four score and ten. It was good immigrant blood which came from Killeleah and Clones in those early days, nor is there yet sign of it running out.

Apprenticeship I

I₁ WAS THE EASTER BREAK; I was to graduate in two months. I was looking for escape from city life, from a big hospital; looking for a place to work where I'd have some backing, yet at the same time be up against real medical problems on my own. It was ten days since I had read the advertisement on the noticeboard at McGill, and here I was in Wakefield, to be interviewed by Dr. Stevenson. When I arrived that Easter Saturday morning, I was met at the station by a young girl. "Are you the new Doctor?" she asked. "Yes, I suppose I am!" I answered. "Daddy's been away all night; I came to get you." We went across the road to *The Maples* where I saw, for the first time, the fireplace set ready to light, the couch in front of it. "The Doctor crossed the river in the night; he's on his way back and should not be too long now," said Mrs. Stevenson. I was left sitting, wondering how he had crossed the river, for I had seen the state of the ice from the train window; weighed down on each bank by open water, the ice cracked along the centre with a definite slope to climb, and open water for ten feet along each edge; quite a feat to cross even on the hard frozen winter road in the centre. In places there were open holes in mid stream; one would have to be careful to keep to the road.

It was not long before I heard rather a heavy tread coming from the kitchen area. With a wide welcoming smile, the Doctor came towards me with somewhat of a nautical, wide stance stride. He was a smallish man, with signs of having lost weight of late. Dressed in grey, with a lighter grey vest, a stand-up wide-open collar and large grey-blue tie. His silvery white hair was long and wavy, and worn straight on end, a grey moustache closely cropped. Hazel flecked eyes, deep set, with dark over-arching brows, gave him a questioning surprised look. His eyes were steady and piercing, though humorous. He held his head thrown back as though he were looking through and far beyond for some sign, something not easily seen at first glance. His nose was large and straight, his jaw, notably square and determined. He was evidently not one to trifle with, not one to lie to. His ruddy face looked tough and healthy; wind and weather had left permanent marks. I was shaking hands with my Preceptor, Dr. Hans Stevenson.

Soon he was on his couch with a hot drink; I, in a great padded armchair. "How did you get across the river?" I asked finally. "Built a plank bridge out to the ice and walked across. The winter road is safe enough, especially at night on the frost, but you must not step off it; you'd go down. The man met me with his team on the other side. He'd built another plank bridge ready for me. In the daytime with the hot sun, the ice is not so safe of course. But I made it all right once more;" and he chuckled. We chatted easily until it was dinnertime at last. Mrs. Stevenson sat at the head of the table; too often the Doctor was called from the meal, if he was there at all, to make it possible for him to preside, she explained. He made a practice of leaving the table to answer the door or telephone, and to rid himself of the patient in an effort to have a quiet meal at his ease.

Besides his wife, there was his sister, "Aunt Mary-Ma" to the seven youngsters as they grew up, one son Bill—aged fifteen, home from high school, four girls—one home from teaching in Montreal, one from Home Economics at MacDonald College— and two younger ones. The two eldest girls were in British Columbia, the eldest married, the second, living with her and teaching music. I was the ninth at the table.

After the meal the Doctor took me to see some patients with whooping cough. With mud coats and felt hats well drawn down over our ears and eyes, we started with a spirited team of small horses. Stella, a bay, made as though she'd eat up and trample anyone who went into her loose box, unless he had a bridle in his hand. She jammed her nose into the bridle, so anxious she was to take to the road. Buster was black, and was possibly the favourite; he had grown up in the family, a pet, spoiled a bit, and he slacked all he could, letting his partner do the pulling. The Doctor, whip in hand, kept reminding him to do his share. Buster would playfully shake his head, tighten up his traces, and do his share for a while. Our first stop was to be at the blacksmith's, to have the top of the covered buggy removed. "It holds the horses back, catches the wind," he said.

We drove through the village, along the Gatineau, here widened out into a considerable expanse; mud flying in places, deep mud puddles, in places patches of ice, it was a dirty drive; past the general store, the farmers' and commercial travellers' hotel, then the Presbyterian church, a second store, then the second hotel, both hotels "dry," (except for bootleggers) largely the Doctor's doing some ten years back. Next we passed the coffin, coal oil and general hardware merchant, then the busy summer hotel, where the proprietress actually went to California for the winter. Then came the long crooked slope up onto the plateau overlooking the village, between bare hedges along the roadside; few cottages, one large winter residence, farmland overlooking the narrow evergreen valleys, clumps of leafless hardwoods; up to the rocky hilltops, where pine and spruce somehow managed to cling. Pointing with the whip over to his left, "That's where we all end up, the cemetery."

Down a sandy hill, and at once up the next, we came to a log house overlooking a wide rolling valley of very fertile land. "These are all Browns, White Luke over across the valley, Henry Natch next, round the corner skirting this rock, Roger lives, married to Henry Natch's daughter, and on down the steep crooked hill we come to Mrs. Burton Brown, and across the swamp on higher ground, Big Ned. Beyond them we are to visit Irish Willie's, and beyond them still, through the bush to the last Brown, Black Luke and his children; all Browns. Some of them the best patients I have. I do all I can. God is their Paymaster," he chuckled. "They warned me I'd not be able to drive all the way to Irish Willie's house; the summer road is flooded; we can tie the horses to the fence and walk around the ploughed field; we can't put the horses across it."

There was a narrow two foot wide strip of grass along the fences which gave us footing and made the way possible, but not without gathering up enough weight of mud on each foot to make it difficult to walk. In any case it did not matter, for the kitchen was tracked far and wide with mud. As it happened, the children were very miserable, but none in bed. The vomiting, nose bleeding, coughing, were severe, nor was there anything to stop these distressing symptoms. Pneumonia was never far away, but without toxoid to prevent whooping cough, and without Phenobarbital to moderate the symptoms, we were very helpless. Plainly these people thought the world of the Doctor and his slightest word.

Back across the muddy field to the horses, and the slow drive up and down hill, past neat farm buildings. We came to a very stout woman leaning on the gate. "What shall I do with my cough, Doctor? It's worse at night," said Mrs. Ned. "It's so hard I puke. There's a baby coming too, my ninth!" We drove home slowly, while the setting sun peeped out between the clouds, showing up the ugly "spring spots" making the land look sad, uninviting, even at times threatening. I felt I could not return to the area, even for a short time.

After supper, with the Doctor on his couch, I again in the big armchair, we talked. Gradually I realised I was undergoing a stiff clinical examination. "What are they doing with appendicitis nowadays? Immediate operation or waiting for the interval to wall off the abscess? What is Frankie teaching you in anatomy? Have you seen any diphtheria yet? That's how I lost my finger," holding up his left hand short of an index finger. "Is scarlet fever severe in Montreal? It's milder here now, but tricky."

The Doctor was called out again at four o'clock Sunday morning, but did not waken me to go with him. A four-inch snowfall during the night, and bright sunshine, made Easter morning sparklingly beautiful, dirty underfoot of course, but trees laden with shining snow as we walked to church. The sermon was on the Creation. The Seven Days were, each of them, twenty-four hours. There was no such thing as evolution. If there was there could be no Easter. Darwin was an impostor. I came back to dinner with sadly mixed feelings; a beautiful countryside, a great opportunity to work, depressingly desperate people, a sadly traditional church; but it was a good dinner, on good china, and with good talk. Perhaps the projected afternoon trip to see an old patient would be somewhat better.

With a lively fresh team we set out; warm spring breezes stirred the dead grasses, a bright sun shone in a deep blue sky, with masses of great cloud. Hillsides were sombre with pines and cedars with their drooping branches, hardwoods with buds almost ready to burst, last year's sumac cones red against the velvety brown stems; everything conspired to enchant. The thought nagged: if only it were not for the people.

All the time, the Doctor's grave, quiet voice told of his work; his means of getting about the country roads; river crossings; snow and ice; storms and hot weather; and scows and bridges; horse problems; rural telephone lines; and all about his daily doings and cases, cases, cases! He spoke of table top drainage of appendiceal abscesses; of suturing a pregnant woman's abdomen, gored by a bull; maternity cases, complicated and difficult; with no help; low beds; poor lighting; but remarkable results in spite of everything.

Then we made a call at Bob T's home, fine farm buildings, an old log house and a wide, very muddy farm yard, a few planks here and there in the worst places. He was an uncouth big man, slow of speech, and clumsy of gait and movement. However, kindly at all times, willing to help out, devoted to the Doctor, Bob was typical of his time, his place and his occupation. "Me mother is sick. Took bad round midnight sudden like. Pain in her side, coughing and spitting blood. Her breath comes short and it hurts. She's eighty five!" I was introduced as a young doctor, a nephew of Mrs. White's! Looking up, the spotlessly clean old lady with vivid Irish blue eyes and wrinkled face, between gasps, questioned, "The first Mrs. White, or the second Mrs. White?" When she was told, "the second Mrs. White", a cloud of disappointment and disinterest came over her. It was very evident that the minister's second wife was not as popular as the first one.

I was more and more depressed. What people! Could I make up my mind to stay and work among them? Would I come back? Could I? Stepping across the muddy yard, stepping from plank to plank, hitching the horses back on the buggy, a great silence grew as we started home. The slanting setting sun threw long shadows, lit up patches of snow on the hillsides across the valley. The Doctor was silent. I had nothing to say. The first mile was over with not a word spoken. Evening lights began to appear in the windows, mud and water flew from the horses' hooves, not a word was said!

Finally half way home, with a sudden turn of the head that I was to get to know so well, "Well, are you coming back?" the Doctor questioned. After a long pause, a very half-hearted "yes" was the reluctant answer. "I'll give you $75.00 a month and your keep as well as the use of the rolling stock and drugs. If things go well, I'll make it $100.00." "Very good," I said, "I don't need holidays, I have no interests away from here. I'll stay two years, but you must help me." So the bargain was made, nor was it ever written down. (When the first month was over I got my $100.00 and bought a microscope.)

By June the Doctor's letter came: "Congratulations on your medal! Come as soon as you can. It's 'Blucher or night'." "Be there June 7th to play Blucher to your Wellington," was my answer. On June 5th as I bowed my head to be capped, the desire to be of use in my new way of life opposed the feeling of inadequacy in my heart. Then came the gold medal, Casey Wood's, "for best clinical standing". Next night, at the opening of the new medical building, the Professor of Medicine came up. "I hear that you are going to a country practice. You should not do it. You could get a good internship in our hospital. You're not a finished man. Don't go," he said. "Yet I've said that I would go. I don't want an internship," I replied. "Where are you going? To Dr. Stevenson? I saw him a while ago. You'd better go, he needs you. He won't be here long!" was the rejoinder. Promptly at supper time on the 7th of June I was met at the Wakefield station by Dr. Stevenson's youngest daughter. "Daddy's away on a case. You're to have supper and I am to drive you down to meet him and bring Mama home. Aunt Mary has supper ready."

So the long first night began, June 7 & 8th, 1911; cold to the city-clad youth. At intervals the friendly, neighbourly midwife brought cups of tea, life-saving cups of tea; but the night was long, long, long. About four o'clock in the morning, the baby girl had arrived and the miserably long cold drive home began. Little did I realise that I was laying the pattern of years to come. Dr. Stevenson was quiet. Suddenly, looking at the sky, he remarked, "Four forty, about. I know by Orion. I've watched him for so many years now. Morning coming!"

I crawled into bed, regretting bitterly my coming, afraid of the responsibility, yet seeing the need, the need I might someday supply. Sleep came at once, and I slept until late. The Doctor had already done a good half day's work when, after an early dinner, a long round of visits began; patients, patients, patients, and telephone company matters.

The Doctor had organised a local rural telephone system to satisfy the needs of his practice. Already, although telephones were only twenty-five years old, the district for thirty miles around was pretty well supplied with service.

Horses had to be fed; the farmer simply took them off the buggy and put them to feed. Despite expostulations, the Doctor had to come in for a cup of tea, really a whole meal in this district. At nine thirty at night, from a back road high up in the hills, with the faint glow of city lights away off to the southwest, the Doctor stopped the horses to rest. Looking across the river he said, "Eighty-one years ago, my mother and father took over six hundred acres across there and cleared a farm. My nephew is still on it. I was born there. I came back to practise here because my parents were still there. You'll see it some time soon, I hope." He started the tired horses and did not speak for awhile, thinking of the eighty-one years, perhaps? Or perhaps more of the fifty years to come with his companion in charge of the practice? How would it go with his patients? What would the years bring them? The sun had been bright, there had been lots to do and to think about, I'd met French-speaking habitants, people in need, people I understood. In spite of exhaustion from a sixteen hour day, the world was a brighter place to be in. I could see that I was needed. The days passed quickly, days filled with incidents big and small; Sunday came hot and bright.

About noon came Baptiste. "Girard is sick, sick nearly a week, not as sick as Marie Ange had been last week, but he seems to have trouble breathing." The Doctor said, "I'm afraid, Baptiste, it's diphtheria again, like Marie Ange! She's well? The serum worked well for her. The young Doctor will see him this afternoon!" I set out along the unknown way to the back parishes. An open buggy, mud bespattered, a good fresh team, nevertheless a three-hour drive over hot dry roads up and down the hills; my first real individual responsibility. The story of the long night, the storm, the struggle for the boy's life, with the end in the morning, has been told elsewhere. Failure was hard to take. Driving home in the fresh early morning after the storm, fog rising from sheltered valleys, a beautiful world, but desolate. Girard was dead; the first great responsibility, and failure. It was many a day, many a year, before such things could be taken in stride. Was there something else that could be done? Could someone else have done better? There was no one else.

Gradually, as time went on, the process of self examination became a habit. If I could not find fault with myself, fault with my methods, then all was well in spite of results. If I could blame myself, the sky was dark indeed. Each day brought its problems. There was the gasping, vomiting, semi-conscious patient, haemorrhaging, soaking the mattress; my call to the Old Doctor for help. But by the time he'd crossed the river, the digital curettage was successful, and the patient in good shape when he arrived. Fresh wild strawberry jam and homemade bread for supper served to revive my discouragement.

Two weeks later, the first forceps case loomed. The Old Doctor was again called to help, but I did my first forceps delivery with his moral backing. Then rumours took a hand: "The Young Doctor doesn't know his work. He had to call the Old Doctor to help him. He's called for help twice since he came. He's no good. He'll never fill the old man's shoes. He's lost his first patient. He nearly lost the haemorrhage case. He couldn't deliver the other baby." Meantime, things had been going faster and faster; sixteen babies in the first six weeks for me. "Do you ever have anything else?" I asked my Preceptor.

Rumour came again, "Mrs. George would have the Old Man in August for her second baby; she'd nearly died the first time. Without him she'd surely die this time." I examined my methods, sat in judgment on myself; decided I was unjustly blamed, and resolved that never again would I call for help. The people would take what I could give them. Brave resolve, for that very day Mme Théophile had a post partum haemorrhage. Five o'clock in the morning, the tenth baby, the wooden spool bed was big, wide and heavy, its foot up on two chairs. Total collapse of the bed and the patient rolled out on the floor; I was not a little discomfited, but when back home for breakfast, and recounting the experience to the Old Doctor, his eyes twinkled, "Golly, I'm glad other people have trouble besides me," he chuckled.

GVHSIB 002228-003

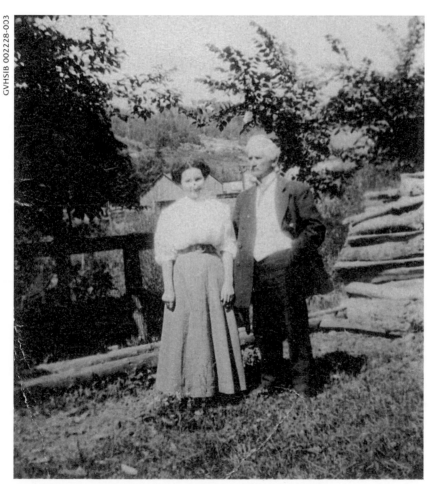

Dorothy Stevenson with her father, Dr. Hans Stevenson. 1909.

Old Joshua

AT TIMES THE CALLS were so distant and so remote we travelled together, my Preceptor happy to take the reins and have the company. We argued good naturedly but earnestly as we drove. "No, no, I can't agree with you," I said, "we're not all mere pawns in the game, to be used and cast aside when the game is done." The level, grave voice came to me through the darkness, "Not all pawns, some kings, some queens, some knights, and some pawns, but each with his many or few moves, straight or crooked, short or long, right up to the inevitable end. That's what I mean; our path is laid out for us, each of us following along. Freedom, there is none." In silence we drove along under the moonless star-filled sky; each star distinct, remote, fixed in its deep blue mystery. In spite of my protest, looking at the fixity of the sky, I almost agreed with the Doctor. "My way has not been the result of a deliberate choice at any point in my life," he went on, "each step has inevitably followed from the previous one, and has inevitably led on to the next. I'm sure we have no freedom; we only follow on."

Again, the expressive silence fell, giving me time for thought, broken only by the cheerful tinkling of the sleigh bells, and the measured quick tread of the almost galloping horses on the crisp snow. Shadowy hillsides dotted with ghost-like snow-laden evergreens, gave a melancholy tone to my thoughts, and perhaps tinged those of my companion. Far up overhead wheeled the Great Dipper, wheeled in endless circles about the Pole Star, following its beaten path.

Suddenly, from the zenith to the horizon slid a shooting star. Nature herself seemed to confirm his opinions. "One thirty," said the Doctor, looking up at the Dipper, "I've watched him many a year, and I know just about where he should be at any time of the night; he's great company."

GVHSIB 02228-004

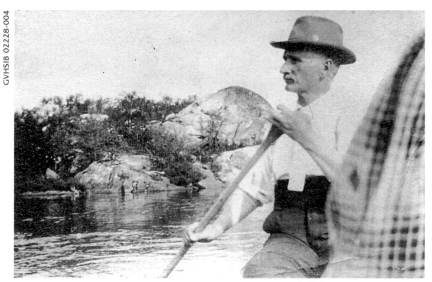

Dr. Hans Stevenson relaxing at the lake. 1911.

The road led down a steep rocky hill, out onto the broad frozen surface of Lac La Blanche. The horses put their best foot forward, encouraged by the unusually level road, and made alert by their unerring instinct for danger, and by the ominous cracking and booming of the ice under the influence of the extreme cold. With ears erect, and smoking breath freezing to their black coats, they scurried along, ever and again turning back one ear to catch the Doctor's encouraging words. "It's all right Gentle. Don't worry Darkie, we'll soon be over it. The ice is good; no danger this time of the year," and visibly the intelligent animals settled into their steady stride.

All around loomed the dark forms of rocky hills, now far, now near, as we hurried along by the irregularities of the shore. Now and again, far off, a night light streamed steadily from some window in a log house, reminding one of the human problems, the comforts and the joys centred about each light. Now and again a barking dog broke the silence of the night, and, waking his master, made him turn over and listen. Recognising the sleigh bells, he wondered at the Doctor's destination on such a cold night. "C'est le Docteur. Ou va-t-il par un temps si froid? Pauvre homme." Then, the miles passing, the lake was left behind, and again the road began its interminable ups and downs, zigzagging amongst the hills, each moment displaying some new shape or shadow. In a reminiscent tone, almost without addressing me, the Doctor spoke.

"Years ago, when I'd first come back to this country, on a night like this, though without the snow to give its uncertain light, on a dark cold star-filled night in late November, I was called to see old Martha. Young Joshua met me at the river, and in a boat half filled with ice, through the heavy cold water, he pulled me over. Then in his old buckboard he drove me slowly up that interminable hill we sped down tonight so easily.

"He spoke in the slow, half articulate way of our mountain people, as we crossed the boulder strewn pasture land where his father's axe had years before felled the first growth of giant pines and left, to the slow decay of years, the stumps we were trying to avoid in the darkness. Winding our way between them, we reached the top of the descent, into the crater like hollow which old Joshua had found and fancied in his youth. Like an old lake bottom it was, fertile and well watered by the never failing stream that drained its gentle slopes, giving rich returns for his labours."

Dr. Stevenson continued, "I remembered old Joshua from my childhood. His visits, to our farms, lasting a week or several weeks were looked forward to with interest and eagerness, at least by the younger generation. We knew his visits meant new boots, and that in making them, we would come very close to a man who, in our childish minds, had done a very dreadful thing. Then his stories of 'Upper Canadie' would introduce us to that very big shadowy world of which we knew so little. It was not until I returned to work among my people, that I learned, little by little, Joshua's story. He had left his well settled Ontario village where he was a cobbler and harness maker, to come north into our tumbled wilderness of hills. No neighbours within a league were there, nor did Joshua care, but it rankled in the breast of Joshua's wife, Mary. Many a time Mary complained of the loneliness; of the rocks about her, and bemoaned her fate. Then, wild with drink, Joshua drove her out into the night, carrying her baby and leading her older children through the snow and the swamps to the far-off shelter of the next neighbour. But Mary's time was not yet come; nor did it come until November. The grim sadness of the listless winds with their burden of cold rain, the melancholy fall of leaf on leaf revealing nakedness of trees and rocks, seemed to enter into her soul, and stir in her a revolt against her lot.

"Joshua, drinking with his cronies, began his interminable wrangling. Mary, the better to conceal her purpose, kept her clacking tongue to herself; but when Joshua and his friends were far gone, late at night, Mary stole away, taking her children with her. Early next morning, when the pale light of early dawn began to break over his encircling hills, Joshua awoke to a fire long gone out, and the less surprising, because half expected, absence of Mary. Fire kindled, courage whipped up with the remains of the night's drinking, cronies gone, Joshua slept far into the day. Night came, but with it no Mary. Winter came and went and still no Mary. Glad to be rid of her, or not caring one way or the other, Joshua lived on alone. Mary, within easy reach in the city, never again saw Joshua or the rocky retreat she hated.

"Mary's sister, Martha, dragged out her existence with Andrew, her husband, not many miles away. Their lives together had been full of misery and disappointment, and after many years Andrew died. Martha was left, childless, to get along as best she could in her log cabin among the piled up boulders and stumps that testified to the periodic half-hearted attempts of Andrew to gain a living from his land. Gradually Martha and Joshua drifted together, neither of them young, neither of them old, both isolated from neighbours, more by the mental and social barrier erected about them by the conscience of our world, for their union was sanctioned neither by Church nor State. As time went on Joshua became more contented, less and less was the bottle the source of discord, more and more he became a steady necessary workman among us. The passing years brought more mature minds, more practical if less strict customs; Martha and Joshua were looked upon as man and wife, as in fact they were, and their sons, young Joshua and his older brother John were in school.

"Many years passed, and as I now recall that stooped, incredibly wrinkled old woman that Martha became, and that shuffling round shouldered figure of a man that was Joshua, I wonder how much freedom of choice they had in shaping their lives.

"That November night comes back to me again, for it was the last time I saw old Martha alive. After months of drying up, the time had come when the wasted old body could not contain the beautiful old soul she had become. With tenderness Joshua had cared for her, and with thankfulness had she accepted his help as her strength failed more and more. On this last night, as I left him standing in his open

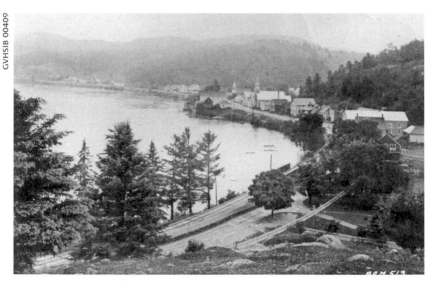

GVHSIB 00409

Wakefield Village, c.1900.

doorway, the dim lamplight lighting up the rugged old face, making his sad Irish eyes shine with their tears, he read my thoughts and jerked out, 'I'se'll be missin' the old 'ooman, she's been good to I. She liked ye Doctor. How'll I thole (endure) it?' That winter, as I was driving, I saw old Joshua jogging along ahead of me, bent forward almost to falling like the very old always are, Glengarry bonnet on his head, wisps of grey hair and shaggy beard blowing in the stray March breeze. Stopping, I picked him up, and after many an enquiry and many a halting answer, he drifted back to the November night when we said goodbye to Martha. 'I'se more content in the ole house where the ole 'ooman was with me. I canna thole living wi' young Joshua. I'se lonesome for the ole 'ooman.'

"Two days later young Joshua came to me. 'My father's poisoned hisself,' he jerked out. There he lay in the old house, in the same old bed where I last saw Martha. On the corner of his neglected cobbler's bench was a saucer of Paris Green within reach of his hand. Bending over him I could almost imagine I heard his last words to me; 'I'se lonesome for the ole 'ooman.' As I bent, I noticed a thin trickle from the corner of his dead mouth, tinged green. Quietly I wiped away the telltale stream, determined to still gossip. 'It's not poison. There is no evidence in favour of it,' I insisted. As if to vindicate my statement, my eyes fell on the swollen body of a rat, lying dead under the table where Joshua had put a crust, green with poison. 'Death is due to lonesomeness,' I said. Wondering at the strange path he had come, I came away."

Early morning was breaking when the horses drew up to the stable door. "You make the road shorter," the Doctor said, as I offered to tend the horses and let him go to rest. However, I was just settling to sleep when came another call, another problem. As I led out fresh horses, I wondered: "Is there any choice, any freedom?"

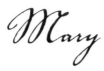

Mary

My Preceptor and I had been up to a mountainside shack, filthy, airless and dark. It was a new baby to a tuberculous mother, five others already; she and her baby probably would soon die from the disease, helped on by lack of food and general misery. Nature, so careful of the race, giving the dying woman strength to bring into the world one more baby before the usual rapid decline. A small feed of standing green oats was all the horses had had, and horses have to eat. We stopped at Mary's hotel on the way home.

My Preceptor was an honoured guest there. Seating him at the head of the table, Mary served him trout, done to a turn, boiled new potatoes, and freshly made wild strawberry jam with homemade bread and new butter for dessert. As for me, I was put far down the table 'below the salt', and served hard fried salt pork, cold fried potatoes, a slab of sole leather apple pie, and boiled tea. Nothing was too good for the Doctor, anything was good enough for the other fellow. We went home laughing, but I was hungry.

The next week on a hot afternoon, the drive down from seeing our tuberculous mother seemed very long indeed. Mary was sitting by the doorway, every inch of her full of misery. Hoping to avoid her, fearing another meal, I bowed shortly as I passed. Suddenly she stood up, beckoning me to stop. "Dang it all, can ye pull me tooth, without breaking it neither?" I was caught. Standing behind her on the sunlit verandah, to my great relief, I found her tooth so loose that had she opened her mouth in the face of a March wind, it might well have been blown down her throat. One yank, and out it came. "Dang it all! Ye did that well. Ye hurted me too, so what ye did, but ye couldn't help it. Here's y'r fifty cints." I felt I was coming up in the world.

June 1911 — My second month in practice

IT WAS A HOT SUMMER DAY. The raspberries were at their best—big, juicy, and sweet. The lake was shimmering in the afternoon heat, inviting in its blue, cool depths. The horses were contentedly munching newly mown green oats, and thereby laying up for themselves a bad attack of colic. Hard driving horses need dry, hard oats, not green oat straw.

It was her first baby. There was no pituitrin in those days to induce labour, only the uncertain use of hot enemas, castor oil, and quinine. One had to wait, and I had already waited one night and one morning. The fried salt pork, boiled potatoes, and well boiled green tea were beginning to pall on me. The berries and a swim seemed indicated, and did help to put in the afternoon.

Long summer evening followed long summer afternoon; but by now the contractions were coming more and more regularly, and made the midwife, this time the patient's own mother, hover threateningly. "Have you taken your nine grains? That always makes it easier." Nine grains of wheat—the old women had great faith in wheat! Midnight brought hard frequent contractions.

"Don't put your arms above your head," directed the midwife mother. "It's bad for you! It will give you beau mal," and later on, "keep your arms down. Yell! Yell all you can! It always does good!" I hung off, reluctant to try forceps for the second time in the month. Forceps, we had been advised to leave at home, so that we'd have to send for them, and by the time they arrived the baby would have come spontaneously, or so said our obstetrics professor. "You will not need them." How far from reality do the great ones of the earth live? How far from us, the ordinary workmen? Reluctantly, I planned to get out the forceps.

Two weeks before, a couple of miles up the lake, on a hot Sunday afternoon, I had, for the first time in my life, used forceps! I had seen them used in hospital. I had admired their ingenious shape and workmanship. I had noted with awe the dexterity of the professor with his anaesthetist, his first and second sterile nurses, his two or three unsterile nurses and his special nurse waiting to give her whole attention to the baby. I had admired the sterile drapes, spotless basin, the sterile instruments; all went together to make a perfect operation.

I had noted all this, but I was alone this early morning on the lakeside with only the grandmother midwife and a couple of neighbours—novices. Somehow I must get rid of the formidable midwife, get her out of the way! I preferred the neighbours, since I felt that I had reason to fear the midwife.

"Would you put some wood in the stove, Madame," I said innocently, hoping thereby to get my forceps ready, unnoticed. "I will be needing a lot of hot water later!" Perhaps there was no wood ready nearer than the far side of the lake, and I might get through before she was back. "Have you finished your bread baking, Madame?"

I had seen a hutch, or dough box, full of bread rising, and ready for baking in the morning. The kitchen had been kept hotter than usual all night and I hoped that the bread had risen enough to need punching down; perhaps even to be put into pans. I might get fairly well through before she caught on. The old lady was, however, getting suspicious. She did not mean to miss the worst.

"Have you fed the hens yet, Madame?" The cock was crowing to the rising sun. I hoped that the hint was not too broad, but off she flounced and I heard the preparations of the hen feed— banging of pails, pouring of milk, pumping water, calling the hens and their chickens; and then the same noises down by the pig pen. All was music to my ears as I rushed the preparations.

Leg braces, scrub up, antiseptic solutions, towels and steaming hot forceps, were ready. The anaesthetic was started, the forceps applied, "left hand, left blade, left side of the pelvis, and left side of the head", and with the instruments articulated, the slow traction began. Release pressure; allow the brain a chance to respond.

At last the head was crowning, the neighbour women were all eyes, tears were dripping down cheeks, and chloroform was dripping onto the mask; a moment more and all would be over, if only Mme S. could delay another minute. However it was not to be!

Back bustled the midwife, back she came like a charging billygoat. She was missing something, I had tricked her! Just as the head crowned, and I was removing the forceps, leaning over my shoulder, the filthy old creature, right from the pigpen, grabbed the head with both hands, and dragged the baby into the world, ripping the perineum, and infecting the whole field. Stormy weeks followed; it was my first infection!

As I write, the mother is a grandmother many times over. Her many children all have families—all but one—for the baby of that morning is a Christian Brother. A woman's sore back, and my memories, are all that remain of that morning by the lake.

La Vie

W<small>ITH AN IMPATIENT</small> "On vous attend, Monsieur le docteur, ça presse!" and grabbing my handbag, the old chap made across a potato field, throwing a breathless word or two of caution over his shoulder as he hurried along. "Prennez garde. V'la le creek! Sautez! Sautez!" But it was too late; I was already sounding the cold depths of the creek, which bounded the lower edge of the potato patch. The temperature of the spring water, and the stickiness of the clay bottom, were fully appreciated long before the warning reached me. The way then led up a grassy slope, with boulders and raspberry bushes scattered haphazard about it, making the ascent more difficult at the breakneck speed we managed to maintain.

Presently we entered the bush, and following a hardly traceable path up the mountain, old Joseph led me on and on, my breath coming shorter as we ascended. Branches brushed across my face, wet with their dew; mosquitoes took their toll, and sang their song behind my ears; roots and stones seemed to conspire to trip me. All around the air was perfumed by the pines and spruce, while the fitful airs of the valley brought up tastes of buckwheat or little gusts of smoke from the chimney in the valley, now far below us. The sailing clouds cast alternate light and shadow on the trees, branches glistening with their dew laden needles, and making an even more varied pattern upon the ground. Still the moon floated on, nearing the horizon, while in the east, pale glimmerings of yellow light told whence the day would come.

Now, near the summit, the trees began to fail, berry bushes succeeded in ripping one's clothes with their wicked thorns. Still the old man led me on with a curious jog trot, sort of a hobble. Down a slope thick with blackberry canes and burr-bearing weeds, we came out into a grain field, around a clumps of trees, and there, by the side of a gleaming lake, stood an old ramshackle log cabin. Long ago, the orderly whitewash on the walls had vanished, and the grouting had fallen from the cracks between the logs. The shingles on the roof had wrinkled and dried in the burning summer sun, except where mosses grew in the shadow cast by the luxuriant growth of hops. Beyond the cottage, and separating it from the rising wooded hills, lay the long narrow shallow lake, in which loons awakened the echoes with their strangely human cry.

From the cabin window shone a feeble light, and from the chimney, a thin white smoke rose and hung in the light mistiness about the roof, and streamed out over the lake. The door opened as we approached, and a woman appeared, talking in a loud rough excited tone: "Oh mon Dieu! C'est trop tard. What it is to live so far in the bush; one can't get a doctor if one is dying. Thank God it's over, but where she'll get the food to feed it I don't know. Her husband is just expected home from the asylum, and he's made nothing for a long time." Meanwhile, going in, I groped about in the semi darkness of the smoky lantern light, stumbled to the stairway, steep as a ladder, and staggered up, striking my head on the floor above as I went. Calling for a lamp, I waited while a hubbub of argument and preparation went on downstairs. At last a tolerable lamp was brought by a girl of some twenty years. She had short, straight, coarse, red hair, everted lower eyelids, flat nose with wide animal-like nostrils, stupid gaping mouth; clearly she was retarded. She was voluble in excuses and reproaches. "Lantern light is good enough for a doctor. What does a doctor want here anyway? There's nothing to do. The little one has come. It is there."

Looking, I saw, in a trunk in front of me, the newborn baby rolled up and muffled as any papoose ever was in a wigwam, dressed coarsely and too warmly, hideous, shockingly so, with its double harelip. "It's a girl, it's my niece," giggled the red-headed girl at my elbow, and, as she spoke, I saw the unmistakable family resemblance; aunt and niece. Turning then to the bed, I saw, lying happy and smiling and uncomplaining, the mother, the faint family likeness clearly traceable, but with auburn hair, fair white skin, well formed nose and mouth, and with pale blue eyes distinctly vacant. By her motioning to her lips and ears, I realised she was a deaf mute, oblivious of her state and station in life, with her erratic mother, retarded sister, insane husband, and now, a deformed baby. God had been good! Amid trouble and turmoil of stress of family life and affliction, He had sealed the ears and stilled the lips, and shut out from the brain all but happiness, a happiness of some inner life that no one could ever break in upon. "God has shown pity," her mother said, "Il sait que la vie est dure pour nous autres."

When I left, the sun was just rising over the bluff hanging over the lake, birds were singing, the soft mists were disappearing, and the morning air was warming quickly under the strengthening of the summer sun. A partridge scurried from the path; the world was awake. Lost in thought, I watched the ground before me. My eyes were arrested by old Joseph's feet, wobbling on ahead of me; they were both clubbed. "C'est ma nièce, voyez vous!" he was saying.

Black and huge above the skyline; looking down upon the fields, looking across them to the hills; standing pointing upwards, pointing eastward and westward; looking northward and southward; warming, comforting, soothing, enlightening the land and its people, stood the Wayside Cross, giving pause to the hurrying thoughts of the roadway. "Yea, tho' I take the wings of the morning, and fly to the uttermost parts of the earth, Thou art there."

Account book entries show that the doctors were often paid "in-kind"—oats, hay, peas, eggs, meat, pasturage, veterinarian service, a buggy, and a horse.

Apprenticeship 11

AUGUST CAME; DOCTOR STEVENSON was away resting at camp. I was in charge with one team and a single horse. The rapidly progressing diphtheria epidemic raged twenty to thirty miles away; extra horses had to be rented.

Twenty-four hours with no let up; Mrs. George reluctantly had to accept the services of the Young Doctor. The patient afraid of me, the strange nurse afraid of me, the husband suspicious, and I more afraid than any of them; but at the end of a long hot day with a late afternoon forceps delivery of a vigorous girl, somewhat of a triumphal home coming for supper, work well done.

The next Sunday was the same thing again. The Old Doctor was expected; I came instead in the fresh early morning; politely received of course, but as the day wore on, more and more evidence of displeasure, of suspicion, of doubt. "Le vieux devait venir. We will go and get him."

"Si vous partez le chercher, je pars moi-même. I know what I can do, I can do what is necessary." It was a big bluff of course, for I longed very much for help, but for the good of my practice, for the good of the district, I had to go through with the case by myself. I could not stand any more grassroots criticism. By sunset, a ten pound boy rewarded my efforts. The sunset over Phillip's Lake was unforgettably bright that night, in spite of fatigue.

From the end of August, things began to improve. The Old Doctor being home again helped a lot. When I handed over a nice big roll of bills from the month's work, his eyes sparkled. "Golly, it's the only job a man can leave behind for a month, and come home to a pile of money!" Early the next morning when the phone rang and I was getting out of the door to the waiting horses, the Old Doctor, in the doorway, watch in hand, exclaimed: "Twenty-three minutes since the phone rang. You'll have to do better than that. Get your bag and your clothes all ready at bedtime. Don't wait for the cup of tea; you can always hold on; the patient can't."

September days; harvest times are soft, but the work did not slacken; maternity, pneumonia, scarlet fever, diphtheria. Two little Indian boys were alone in the bush hunting; the front of a thigh was shot away, and after lying in a shack for a week, far off the beaten track, the child was carried out on a stretcher, leg splinted with maple leaves for padding. The runaway of a farm team resulting in a lad with a ruptured urethra; the days were full. I was on my way home after a long wet, cold day, with twelve miles to go, and three children to share a meagre 15,000 units of diphtheria serum. At supper, after nine o'clock, I reported to Dr. Stevenson. "Not enough serum; best take the other team and go back and give them more," was his response. That was a bad night. The mother was surprised to hear my knock after midnight!

Winter was coming early. It was November the third, with iron-hard, frozen ground, scant snow, but a bright sun. A call to Black Joe's—'the young'uns be pukin'. "Min, come for a drive," Dr. Stevenson said to his wife. "Don't go, Hans, let Harold go. Stay at home and rest." So I went, five miles up and down hills, to where Black Joe himself sat in front of his shack, whittling a chip in the sunshine. One of the two 'young 'uns' came too close. "Get out o'me way, ye young scat. If ye don't get outa me way, I'll carve the hearts out of yez." Two other children were stretched out on chairs; one needed two chairs, and one needed three. They had finished 'pukin'; the trip was useless in every way.

The Old Doctor could not stay still, so that shortly after I had left he said, "Come on Min, we'll go and see if we can get some wood from the mill man. Besides, I want to try out the colts." They had just got back and we walked together from the stable where the horses rested up for the next trip. "It must be the help I've had this summer!" he said. "I feel fine; you should buy me out. Things are going well. I'll do what I can in the office while you do

GVHSIB 00366

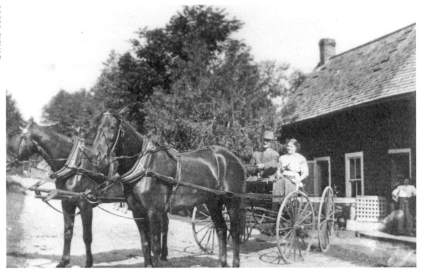

Dr. Hans Stevenson and his team on a housecall.

the driving; think it over. When you are away I'll take the odd run."
After supper, the Doctor's sisters came in for the evening. Lying
on his couch by the fire he read aloud to all. Bedtime came and I
got no chance for a conference.

Four o'clock in the morning; the clip-clop of horses hooves
on the road woke me. The horses stopped, and the bell rang. "Me
'ooman's taking fits! Come quick."

"Is she expecting a baby?"

"Yes, not for a few days though."

So short was the preparation for leaving the house that I did
not leave the usual note as to my destination. My first *eclamptic*
(toxaemia of pregnancy); totally unconscious she was, tongue
transfixed by her one upper tooth, enormously fat and lying on a
feather mattress.

Three hours later, after administering sweat baths and
sedatives to my patient, I received the news.

The Old Doctor had died an hour before. Leaving a colleague,
Dr.Pritchard, in charge of my patient, I drove slowly home,
drove home with shoulders bowed under a weight I felt beyond

my endurance. It was winter three days later when we buried him. The parson's sermon was on survival after death.

Today, after fifty years, now old in turn, I still hear of the Old Doctor. He survives in his doings, doings for his patients. His works do follow him.

~

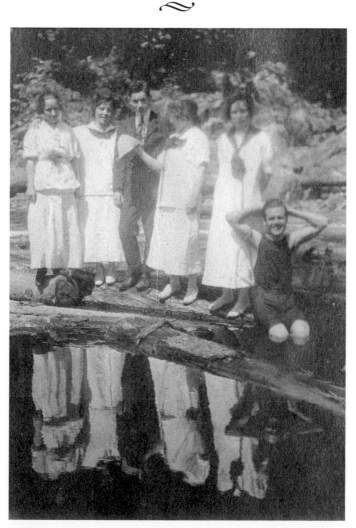

Stevenson family: Betty, Dorothy, Bill, Maddie, Ruth and friend. 1910.

Critical Acclaim

THE IRISH PRETENCE AND AIRS, and the Irish eloquence, have always interested me. Here, in a new land, the old Irish customs and manners of speech remain unimpaired. John, the incomparable liar, the never-daunted story teller, called down blessings on my head, as we would string beads, first a bright one, then a brighter, and when one is amazed at the turn of speech, a dazzling compliment that would stagger the mere ordinary imagination.

"Shure, your honour, the late Doctor Hans was a great man. Niver a word from his mout' but 'twas full o' wisdom. 'Niver you mind John m' dear fellow,' he said to me, shure he did, 'take care o' your tubes and, you'll be all right.' Well he's gone, the dear man, God rest his soul and give him peace, and you're here to do his work, and carry it on, whatsoever it be. Shure he was a foine doctor, but I'm thinkin' his place is well taken. What's the use of having a medical man in the district, that knows all about you as soon as he sets eyes on you, if ye don't go to him when ye be sick? Shure you're the best man about your business I ever see'd. 'Let him alone', I says to Maggie, 'That man knows his business.' 'Tom,' says he, 'won't last past six o'clock', and be damned if he did yer honour, and you know what's the right thing to do too, yer honour, for, says you, 'Git the priest for that man right away,' says you, you did, 'for he may go onny minute.' Shure enough, come six o'clock, says he 'John, I'm dying.' 'Sure you are,' says I, 'and you can't help it neither, for the doctor said it,' and with that he turned and was away in a minute. That's what I call a foine doctor, yer honour, to get the priest, and see after the man's soul and all."

And all the time, the dirty old rapscallion laid stress on this or that passage with his hands, his voice changing almost as though two people were holding a heated conversation, and, looking at his dirty person, my mind, pictured the log hut up on

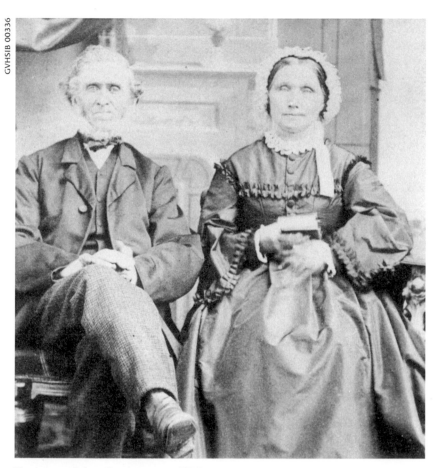

GVHSIB 00336

Thomas and Ann Stevenson, c.1890.

the clay hills where John and his brood of pretentious children lived, dirty, ignorant of any books, deceitful, double-dealing, but with the airs of duchesses. And still the old chap wandered on with his endless measure of praise and blessings, 'til in sheer desperation, I did what he wished—for nothing—and he left me wondering how long I could be spared a similar consultation.

The Years Between 1

THE YEARS BETWEEN BEGAN November the 4th, 1911, the moment the Old Doctor died, leaving me with his heavy burden. There was a good deal of medical work to do at the time, and there were the Doctor's books to post, bills to get out, accounts to collect; too many of them. There were accounts to pay; a very few. Within a fortnight I was held responsible for the collection of all the accounts, accounts running back possibly twenty or more years. In three weeks my patients were all better, afraid of me, or dead; no patients left, no work, no money. There were five horses, three cutters for the winter, three buggies for the summer, a sulky, a dump cart, a quantity of feed, a stock of drugs; all to dispose of, or for me to buy and use. I could not easily pick up and leave everything hanging. But I had no work to do to make money, nor money to pull out with. Nevertheless I bought the running gear and drugs for eight hundred dollars; my mother's money, but the horses still had to be fed.

Christmas was coming; and with Christmas, the Doctor's second daughter, in spite of herself, began to impress me. I had heard a lot about her during my five months with her father; her music, her swimming, her tennis. I had taken a dislike to her without waiting to meet her. She returned from Vancouver on November 9th, 1911, resenting the presence of her father's replacement.

One very muddy November day, wet and cold, she insisted on coming for a drive with me despite my unwillingness to take her. It was her father's horse; she was determined to come, she told me later. I began to notice her. By December 27th, I was lost, but she gave me no encouragement. I was in despair; no hope, in debt, and no work. She was leaving for Vancouver in a few days. It was New Year's Day; bright sun, cold, good snow roads. With a fresh team, one lone patient, and a big white world to see, and a chance to be beside her for twenty long miles each way. On the way out the sun shone, the horses were wild and flew over the snow. Pine trees were heavy with snow, beech trees full of golden brown leaves rustling in the breeze; sumac cones red against the sparkling snow; and jays with raucous cry, a flash against the blue sky. A crow slowly and croakingly flew across the way, a squirrel gathered tamarack cones; it was a day to be alive and to remember. The way out was bright with talk and chatter and sunshine; the way back, even more swift because the horses were going home, became more and more silent. Not a word was spoken for miles, until finally, not a mile from home, she said, "Perhaps if I got to know you better..." It was enough; my future was settled. We had a good New Year's celebration after all, in spite of few patients, no money and lots of debts.

That drive began all that has mattered since in life. A trip to Vancouver in 1913; a decision not to move west; and marriage in 1914, just after the war began. That drive too, made possible the years between.

(Editor's insert)

The five short months since graduation had been filled beyond understanding with new experiences. There were seemingly impossible situations, but always with the assurance of his Preceptor. Usually he had the consolation that he was doing some good, filling a great need in helping his exhausted mentor as well as a community in great need. There was little time to contemplate, but at the back of his mind was the thought that this was a learning situation. In two years time, he could reconsider, determine whether this was what he wanted to do with the rest of his life and possibly, having saved a small amount, he might be in the position of offering to buy into the secure practice, or to move to another area. One other irritant remained. His parents, well-established in Quebec, owning extensive valuable historic property at Beauport, dreamed aloud of his coming to settle in the community where he had grown up. They were vocal about his needing to take the opportunity to do some post-graduate work, specializing in some aspect of medicine.

The sudden death of Dr. Stevenson in 1911, brought agonizing circumstances. Harold was part of the household and had been for five months, a practical necessity since the phone system remained in the

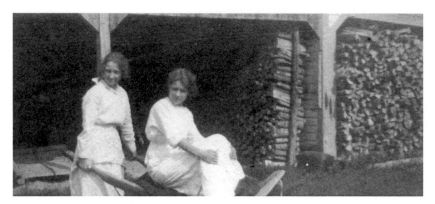

Wood supply at *The Maples*, c.1910.

home and office. It was not the standard home. Three roomy areas on the south side of the residence housed a waiting room, a consulting room, examining room, and dispensary, as well as four separate phones in the hallway to each of the four privately owned and operated telephone services. The practising doctor needed to remain with the office part of the building.

To contribute to the complexity of the household, The Maples *housed the five younger members of the family and their mother, as well as Dr. Stevenson's widowed sister, Mary Stevenson Shouldice, who ruled in the kitchen. This appears to have been a satisfactory arrangement for 'Minnie'— Mrs. Hans Stevenson—allowing her the freedom to occasionally meet her husband with a fresh team of horses as he headed in another direction, or of driving with him. It was not unusual for patients to remain with the family for a meal, while they awaited the return of the doctor.*

The two eldest daughters, Anna, married with a young son, and Ella, living with her in British Columbia, were unable to be with the family. Ella took the train trip alone arriving home after her father's funeral, and remained for two months.

Harold had established himself well with the four younger girls, their brother, and with Mrs. Stevenson, all of whom treated him as a member of the family. But relations were strained with Ella, who, in her grieving state, resented his intrusion into the circle. He, in turn, a sensitive young man, gave her a wide berth. Her music added another dimension to the bereft family, and Harold was drawn into the comfort of this. Little by little the relationship thawed, until, just prior to her proposed leaving, at the beginning of January, he found himself enchanted with this charming, gentle, artistic young woman. Ella had, while living with Jack and Anna McDonald in New Westminster, made a small living by teaching piano, but led a somewhat carefree life to which she seemed determined to return.

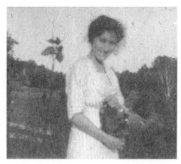

Ella Stevenson, c.1909.

Harold apparently escorted her to the station, but was unable to remain until the train left. The first of many letters reads:

The Maples
Wakefield, Jan. 8/12

My Dear Ella,

I'm not blue yet and you've been gone almost five hours or to be more exact, four hours and fifty-five minutes. The house is very empty all the same and dinner was a dirge—no one said anything much and no one ate much either. … I was watching from the office door for you while the train was at the tank, but two prospective patients came in and I had to follow. One wanted to pay a bill of $3.00—I say, 'wanted to', but truth to tell he wanted not to pay it and said so in the longest way possible, and the train passed on as it usually does except that it took you too. …

Now 'til next time, be happy and busy, as I know I shall be while waiting your first letter which I won't burn except with my green eyes.

Goodbye, Harold

The correspondence continued, with several letters weekly in both directions. In fact, by July, 1912, Ella was writing… "You're the dearest darling boy, I've had a letter every day since Monday and one over.

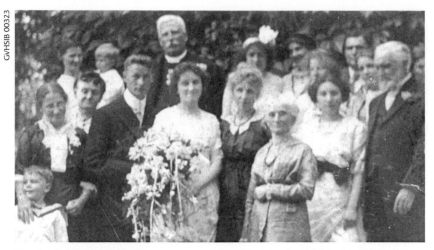

Harold Geggie and Ella Stevenson marry at *The Maples*. 1914. Mrs. James Geggie front, at Harold's elbow Mrs. Hans Stevenson at the bride's left (dark dress), Aunt Mary (front).

You write such sweet nonsense. I like it even if I do know it is not true."

By March, 1913, Harold had approached Ella with the idea of their settling in Quebec City, to which Ella was adamantly opposed. He also was receiving conflicting advice from colleagues, of the difficulty in becoming established in practice in Quebec City, and of the excess of doctors in British Columbia. Finally, despite the expense, which he could ill afford, Harold arranged for a Dr. Aylen (possibly of Aylmer) to do a locum for a month, when he travelled out west to spend time with Ella and to consolidate their plan to marry and settle in Wakefield. Both had determined that they wanted to spend their lives together. Was the final choice of continuing the practice in Wakefield a compromise, or had Harold, in the intervening months, determined that this was where his heart was in medical practice, that these were the people he wanted to serve?

There is little doubt that, despite the long, cold and somewhat perilous drives across uncertain ice-clogged rivers, and impossible roads, and the pressure from his parents; the very values they had instilled in him of responsibility and service, were the determining factors in his remaining in the community which was becoming his home.

❧

The Years Between II

Work began to come my way; after all, the public has a conveniently short memory, and there was no one else within reach. Practice has changed so much over the years—people too have changed. As a background to our thinking, it is necessary to try to draw a picture of the early years.

There was more fatalism long ago: "Le Bon Dieu m'en a donné seize. Il savait bien que je pouvais pas en prendre soin; Il m'en a pris huit, j'en ai huit dans le cimetière—God gave me sixteen children. He knew I couldn't look after them; He took eight, I have eight in the cemetery."—infantile digestive upsets.

"I done the best I could. He wasn't very sick 'til today; I watched him choke."—diphtheria. "There's no feeling too bad for a pregnant woman. Doctors can't help you 'til the last day." There was practically no prenatal care, so we had toxaemias of pregnancy.

"I won't let my mother go to hospital to be butchered," so his mother died with general peritonitis. "Do all you can for her, but I won't have an operation at all,"—a gangrenous gall bladder; she died too. St. Luke's Hospital in Ottawa was known as the "Butcher Shop." There was, of course, some justification for each of these attitudes.

There was, in my practice, almost always an infant dying of digestive troubles in those days, caused by raw unpasteurized milk, heavy with cream or top milk, or Jersey milk. Some melted away after many weeks, some ran a sudden high temperature and were dead in a few days. The death rate was probably one a month; the morbidity frightening.

We never left the house without a supply of diphtheria antitoxin. Often the serum worked miracles. Often given in too small doses or given too late, it was disappointing. Besides, at two dollars a thousand units and many miles to drive, adequate doses could easily wreck both the doctor and patient financially.

There was no way for a doctor to keep office hours; patients driving many miles and waiting many hours, the doctor on the road and driving home again. It is little wonder that the majority of women never saw a doctor until they were in labour. Accidents of pregnancy and labour were bound to happen, meaning a high perinatal death rate for both mother and offspring. Most men married the second time, and said fatalistically: "My wife died when the baby came." The maternal death rate was about one every second year; one in two hundred and sixty, or four per thousand. The causes were placenta praevia or accidental haemorrhage, toxaemia with or without convulsions, and least of all, although too often, puerperal infection.

Surgery has changed so much over the years; it was a brave person who willingly accepted operation; he had to be cornered. Today there are people asking for more or less unnecessary surgery. Doctors have changed. It is hard to estimate the debt the general practitioner owes to specialism; yet the multiple specialties are bewildering. Long ago, a patient with a typical acute appendicitis insisted that I should accompany him to the hospital for the operation; "You never know what them fellows will do when they get youse down there." (His sister had died some months before with a general peritonitis; he's still living.) There have been cases of choosing the wrong, or the insufficiently trained specialist, but the results of surgery today, properly planned by the G.P. and specialist, are astonishingly good, compared to the old days. Improved anaesthetics and anaesthetists, with blood transfusions, intravenous fluids, stomach suction and antibiotics, have contributed much.

From personal experience, surgery in 1925, and surgery in 1947, are worlds apart. More or less calculated risks were taken in 1925, but with a degree of certainty in 1947.

Drugs have changed. In 1911 we had a whole row and alphabet of Tinctures:

Tincture Asafeotida

Tincture Benzoin

Tincture Calumba

Tincture Digitalis

Tincture Ferri Perchlor

Tincture Gentian

Tincture Hyoscyamus

Tincture Juniper

Tincture Kino Co

Tincture Lavender

Tincture Nux vomica

Tincture Opium

Tincture Squills

Tincture Triticum

Tincture Uva Ursi

Tincture Valerian

Tincture Zingiberis

Seventeen bottles in a row, and of all of them only *Tincture Digitalis* today, to add to an old person's cough mixture. The others, and many more, are gone.

Of antispasmodics and tranquillizers, there is a whole row today in various doses. Barbiturates, and the rest, described as slow acting, prolonged acting, fast acting, short acting, habit forming, and non-habit-forming. Today we have a whole shelf of them, a confusion of them. In my early days, the bromides were the only sedatives, in spite of the potential skin and digestive effects.

Of anaesthetics, we had two, the inflammable ether, impossible to use with open fires, oil lamps and wood stoves; or the dangerous chloroform. Chloroform we gave with one hand while we opened abscesses or set bones with the other; with the patient wiggling as the result of a

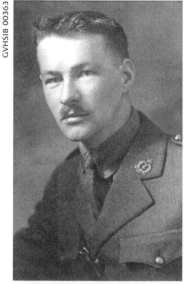

GVHSIB 00363

Capt. Harold Geggie, M.D., c.1918.

light dose for fear of giving too much. We had our trials with chloroform, and it was a wonder what we did with it all the same. One patient, dying with a tuberculous throat, put herself to sleep each night with it for months. A nurse living twenty long snowy miles from me, wrote, "You must fill my chloroform bottle again; you may not be able to get to me in time next month." When I did get to her for her first baby, she was composedly sniffing up chloroform as each pain came. Chloroform was given to a small girl having multiple convulsions with whooping cough, with good results, in spite of pneumonia. A mature woman with severe whooping cough spasms carried a small bottle of chloroform in her belt to use with each bout of coughing. I gave chloroform to quiet the spasms of a terminal tetanus; and chloroform, one in four hundred, made many nasty mixtures tolerable to take. It was a good friend for many a year; it's almost "out" now.

The search was for stimulants in the early days; *Tincture Nux Vomica*—"mixt.alk. with nux" was a frequent stomachic—I made it up in gallon lots. Liquor Strychninae went with hydrochloric acid stomachic. In typhoids and pneumonias, we were always eager to find and try out another new stimulant. Alcohol was considered a stimulant, caffeine sodium benzoate every eight hours, alternated with camphor in oil every eight hours, was used in most typhoids and pneumonias. It was an event of great note when Coramine appeared. A man had done his duty when he prescribed Coramine, after meals and at bedtime; he had gone one better, and nothing else could be expected, when he gave Coramine hypodermically.

Then it was stimulate; now it is more often, sedate, calm and tranquillize. We had quite a few crude drugs; for instance— Quassia chips, Digitalis leaves, Liquorice powder, Rhubarb root, Bitter aloes, Senna leaves, Senna pods, Stramonium leaves, and a drawer full of dried Mullein leaves for asthmatics to smoke.

Most of my evenings at home after supper were taken up with weighing out and folding up countless powders such as "morph. hydrochor. gr. 1/4" for some terminal case of cancer. We had few pills or tablets, fewer capsules. Powders of Antifebrine or the milder Phenacetin, "fever powders" often used to satisfy a fussy mother and let the doctor sleep until morning. They were usually blown up with "pulv. creta. aromat."; they tasted better going down. Some nights it would be Cocoa butter suppositories with Oak galls and pulv. opii; another night, pills of one sort or another; Gum tragacanth and Liquorice powder.

Today, prescribing drugs may be but a game of keeping up with the latest advertisement from some twenty-five companies, each with approximately the same drugs of impossible to remember chemical names, done up in flashy capsules of unearthly color, and called by fanciful company-made names. The druggist or dispensing doctor merely counts out the required number, packages them up and has done his job. Who shall say which system is or was the better, the old or the new? We thought that we were doing good long ago; we sometimes wonder if we are doing good now.

Among the keepsakes on my book shelves are a few texts used by my Preceptor, at McGill, in the 1880s. *Pepper's Systems*, 1885, in five volumes; Austen Flint's, *A Treatise of Medicine* (1873), and Thomas Huxley's, *Lessons in Elementary Physiology* (1885). An hour spent with these old volumes will give a depth to the medical picture for any student as a background to the daily round. I take down an old text and read once again the picture of scarlet fever, or erysipelas, or childbed fever, or malignant sore throat, read them again as Rush saw them or as Pepper met them in the 1870s, even as Osler described them in *Canada Medical Journal* of the 1880s. It is a good excuse to compare these old writings with my personal observations of my early years and today, when most of them have all but disappeared.

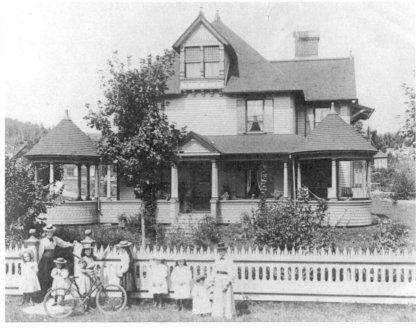

GVHSIB 00307

The Maples, Dr. Hans Stevensons' residence and office, c.1890.

Few modern doctors have ever seen the diseases which kept us on the alert; kept us driving all night and all day in spite of fatigue, hunger and exhaustion, lest we lose a life—diphtheria, pneumonia, typhoid and cellulitis. My first brush with malignant sore throat, or diphtheria, was three days after graduation, twenty-six miles from home; all through the night, with death coming in the early morning for a bright, fair-haired, blue-eyed lad of fourteen. His sister had a mild attack but it was enough for it to spread all over the community, with forty cases, and eleven deaths.

Diphtheria stayed with us all through the years. Never did we stir from the house without the costly serum, even at two dollars a thousand units and needing forty to fifty thousand per patient, enough to cripple doctor and patient financially. Once I attempted to do a tracheotomy with the father and mother assisting, but had to give up when the parents forced me to. The child died soon after and his brother did also in two weeks, for they called me too late. He got up out of bed, where he was to stay for months for cardiac weakness, and dropped in a heap on the floor before he got to the window. And, there was the lad, also, in a filthy home, who died with multiple gangrenous patches over a large area of his body, doubtless diphtheria in his already profuse impetago.

In the late 1870s, at McGill, Dr. Stevenson assisted Dr. Osler with an autopsy on a case of diphtheria. In removing the skull cap, he scratched the first finger of his left hand. This led to diphtheria infection in, and amputation of the finger, followed by generalized peripheral diphtheritic paralysis, and the loss of his year at college. In the course of his practice, my Preceptor had two more diphtheritic infections. He knew diphtheria. "Mal de gorge" always brought a response at any time of the day or night. My last diphtheria case was in 1945; a lad just home from the army of occupation of Holland, and I saw him within the first twenty-four hours of his illness, propped up in bed, strumming a guitar. His throat was heavily coated. There was no change next day in spite of penicillin and antiserum. Two days later he was no longer able to strum. Cardiac paralysis had supervened, general paralysis spread, and he died in three weeks, totally paralysed. I still watch for diphtheria, but of my three colleagues in practice, only my oldest son has seen a real case of it. The year 1959 was the first one in which no deaths from diphtheria occurred in all of Canada. Immunization with toxoid has been effective.

Pneumonia was "the ten days terror", or "the old people's friend", but is no longer; with antibiotics they get better. "Sudden pain in the ribs, cough, spitting blood", always brought us out. There was little of real curative value to give. Early one morning, after a very snowy drive, I found my twenty-four-year-old young giant looking not too sick at all, but the flaring nostrils suggested pneumonia, and when I sat him up to look at his chest, the right lung was solid. Two days more and he was dead.

I walked three miles each way through the bush one spring, to save a twenty-mile drive with horses around by the road, to see a young girl. At last, to save her real final agony, and deciding she might as well die easily, I gave her a quarter of morphine. I walked back through the bush feeling like a murderer, unable to take stock of birdsong, running water, or spring ferns. She had her crisis that night, and is today a grandmother. I got the credit for curing her.

Sixteen days we watched for a crisis; half a dozen private nurses in succession developed "stomach ulcer" trying to cope with the filthy conditions they had to face in one house. Confluent impetago patches covered the patient's body from his filthy mattress. Crisis would not come, neither would death. The last night the nurses were in rebellion. "He should be dead; we won't give him any more stimulants; he should be dead." He did die that night; the Doctor was blamed.

Leo got his crisis on the seventeenth day, and got better, even though he did develop a phlebitis in his left leg and is no doubt still lame wherever he may be. Time and again I telephoned ahead to make sure he was still living before starting out on my daily visit of fifteen miles over spring roads to see him.

Pneumonia always rated a daily visit and at times, where at all possible, several visits a day. "A ten day terror", at times it was even longer. Then in the first year of the war came sulfanilamide (M & B 492). We doled it out carefully, gave soda with it, and dreaded the ones who could not or would not drink. Pneumonia lost its terror.

Whereas, not daring to name it, I called it "congestion" or "a cold on the chest," my son, when he came back from overseas, went happily on his way saying "You've got pneumonia, you'll soon be better," and so they would. With the end of the war in 1945, we began to give penicillin, and the classic picture of pneumonia was no more; a death from this disease in this day of chemotherapy and antibiotics is rare.

The Version

*(A turning procedure to deliver a baby by breech,
used before Caesarean Sections were common.)*

MY INEXPERIENCED SHOULDERS carried the whole load; some of
the prestige of my Preceptor gradually was mine; there were few
doctors in all the country. Moreover, Mary was rooting for me.
"Hadn't he pulled me last tooth? Did it well too, dang it all!" I felt
I had a friend at court. The first snow had fallen in the night. All was
sparkling white and beautiful, but by noon the sun was hot once
more, the roads one long stretch of mud, mud flying from horses'
hooves and buggy wheels—water and more snow and more mud.
I was wearing my mud coat and old slouch hat, both weighed down
with many days' mud—dry and less dry. There was no comfort in
driving twenty-two miles to help out an older doctor.

Mary had no doubt told the "dirty Frenchman" to get help;
it was Mary's territory; the patient, Mary's friend. I felt I would be
on trial; an unknown doctor, a critical Mary, perhaps a hard case;
but perhaps it would be over before my arrival, with the slow-going
bad roads. I almost hoped so—yet—I hoped to prove myself too.
It was a long labour, an arm presentation, an old patient, fifteenth
baby, an incompetent, careless doctor, having more tobacco in his
kit than anything else, and unwashed forceps from his last case,
loosely wrapped in newspaper.

Mary stood over the patient and would not let him proceed;
she stood toothless, muttering, "the dirty bug!" Mary was right,
that's what he was. "Do a version—for God's sake, do a version!
I will do the extraction," he said to me. The version was easy
enough. The two limbs came down in a trice. I surprised myself,
and left the extraction to my colleague as he desired. After all, it
was his case. The bed was low, the Doctor would not go down on
his knees, nor even bend his back. Perforce I had to caution him—

69

my senior in practice by twenty-five years—caution him about his own case!

Finally he delivered a limp girl, blue, and apparently lifeless. No effort was made to resuscitate the baby; she was just thrown on the foot of the bed, while the Doctor mopped his brow, and lit a cigarette, bemoaning his fatigue and sore back. Nothing more for me to do. How I regretted not taking over the case as Mary had asked me. I could not have done worse myself. However, better look over the baby.

Then came hot and cold baths—mouth-to-mouth resuscitation I half imagined that there was a faint heartbeat. So limp, so blue, so congested; minute by eternally long minute passed and there was no response. Back aching, bending back and forth to blow the breath of life into the slack chest, minute after minute, eternity after eternity, it seemed. Sixteen minutes passed, no response. Eighteen minutes and there was still no response—a slight sigh. "Leave it be, won't you; don't interfere with God's doings. He wants it dead!" said my colleague.

Mary was frantic; I was angry, but my back no longer ached; there was life in it. Twenty minutes, and a faint breath.

Last winter, when the patient of that day ended her long life with a failing heart, Mary, her daughter, was anything but a lifeless morsel of humanity. Mary has a hotel in the mining country, like her godmother.

"Dang it all, the dom man breathed intil it. It was flat and dead. He breathed intil it and it lives, he made it live." Mary told every willing listener in shop or bar. My reputation, if not my future, was made that day. Mary was my friend—my slave, from that day out.

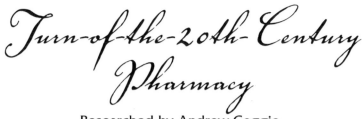

Researched by Andrew Geggie

A GLANCE THROUGH the pharmacological textbooks of the period brings to mind the uncertain chemistry of the medieval alchemist. Turn-of-the-20th-century texts like King's American Dispensatory, by Harvey Wickes Felter, M.D., and John Uri Lloyd, Phr.M., PhD. (1898), or A Compend of Materia Medica, Therapeutics, and Prescription Writing, by Samuel O. L. Potter, M.D. (1902) are instructive, though the reader is urged to keep a Latin grammar handy:

Tincture Asafeotida — a resin used as a stimulant, antispasmodic and expectorant in croup, pertussis, infantile convulsions.

Tincture Benzoin (a Sumatran tree) — used to promote expectoration in chronic diseases of the air-passages, as a dressing for fresh wounds, to improve the taste and odor of other medicines

Tincture Calumba (an African vine) — used in dyspepsia, chronic diarrhoea, and dysentery.

Tincture Digitalis (Foxglove) — used, as today, for weak, rapid, irregular heart action, with low arterial tension.

Tincture Ferri Perchlor — ferric chloride was given for pharyngitis and diphtheria.

Tincture Gentian — a powerful tonic to improve the appetite, strengthen digestion.

Tincture Hyoscyamus (Henbane) — contains alkaloids, including scopolamine, used for nervous irritability.

Tincture Juniper — stimulating, carminative and diuretic.

Tincture Kino Co (Kino is a south-Asian tree) — a mixture of kino, opium, camphor, oil of cloves, cochineal powder, ammonia and alcohol used for diarrhoea and cholera.

Tincture Lavender — a remedy for flatulence, hysteria, gastric uneasiness and nausea.

Tincture Nux Vomica — a source of strychnine, used for atonic states of the gastro-intestinal tract.

Tincture Opium — used in relieving pain and spasm, as a cerebral and spinal stimulant, for rheumatism, neuralgia and gout, for nervous irritability, diarrhoea and dysentery, asthma, colic, cholera, hysteria and tetanus.

Tincture Squills — an irritant, emetic, cathartic, diuretic, and expectorant, used for chronic cough.

Tincture Triticum — this extract of Couch grass was used for urinary tract irritations and 'gravel'.

Tincture Uva Ursi — Bearberry was an astringent urinary tract tonic, also used in chronic diseases of the larynx, bronchial and pulmonary tissues.

Tincture Valerian — a cerebral stimulant used for hysteria and chorea, with mental depression and despondency.

Tincture Zingiberis — Ginger was used for loss of appetite, flatulence and spasmodic gastrointestinal contractions.

Once in a Lifetime

I HAD KNOWN NELLIE AND MICHAEL for many a year as a peculiar old brother and sister who lived just off the beaten track, which served for a short cut from our village to The Corners. In summer, when the woods were green and cool, their little clearance, with its uneven fringe of rocky hills round about, brought pleasant thoughts as one passed. Bright sunshine shone on the white-washed logs of the house, its end covered by Virginia Creeper. Nearby, a luxuriant lilac bush, a ragged garden of pink and white phlox in front of the house, made a pretty picture in late afternoon, with the bluish smoke rising from the chimney and drifting out over the little lake where the ducks rested motionless after the heat of day.

One would see an old woman or an old man standing somewhere near the beehives, by the chicken coop, at the plough, or with the scythe; an old person of uncertain age, dressed in an indescribable medley of fabrics, of patches, of colours, of fashions, giving a human touch to the scene. A wave of the hand, a shout, and they and their home were hidden from view, blotted from the memory, an incident in the daily round. And in the winter, over the hardly beaten track. Because of the drifts, the road led down the gully running between the house and the stable. The frosty air, dry and good, if stinging to the breath, made the smoke rise straight up from their chimney against the blue immensity of the sky. Cattle wandered about from straw stack to straw stack, to the water hole in the lake, breathing out clouds of steaming breath, which, freezing about their heads, gave them, too, a grizzled old-age look.

One got a closer look at the old people in the winter. At this time of year I often stopped to chat with one or other of them, about the roads, the cold, last week's storm, the drifts, and many other little things that go to make up life in our world. Good faces they had, pink, evenly weathered and age-worn; bright blue Irish eyes; greying hair, hard horny hands, feet swathed in rawhide boots, ragged and patched coats padded out with many undergarments. Never, however, did I see them together. Never did one mention the other. They lived by the side of the road in our little world, and as in bigger worlds, they lived their own lives their own way. Big and important to themselves perhaps, a mere episode to the rest of us. Yet they had a story, as I found out later. They had sentiment, romance, feelings; they were very human after all.

One night, Nellie sent me a message by a passerby; Michael was sick and needed me badly. I made the ten miles easily under a deep blue cloudless sky full of stars, lit up on the southeastern horizon by the far-away glow of city lights, to remind us that our problems were as a puff of wind that ruffles the waters of a mountain lake, compared with the long swells of the open ocean.

Michael had been sick for several days, I found; dragging himself out to feed his horses and back again, to sit shivering by the stove, shivering and spitting blood. Nellie seemed to have watched him very closely, for she could tell just how and when he fell sick. But I could not help noticing that she never said a word to him, nor did he give her a look or a word of approval or confirmation such as one might have expected. I thought nothing much about it at the time, and doing what was necessary, I made my way home again, across the snow under the shining stars. The newly risen moon flooded the gullies with light and shadows, making the frosted leafless trees a lacework of jewels against the sky; making the mountain sides glisten above the shadowy sloping pasture lands, dotted here and there by clumps of dark cedars or towering pine trees, laden with their burden of snow and sleet.

For several days, Michael continued unchanged; a little worse, a little weaker, if any change there was at all; the looked-for crisis of pneumonia delayed. Nellie was plainly showing the strain. Day by day, I hated to break the news to her and tell her my secret thoughts. At last, Michael was in despair, and Nellie, in the deepest depths, followed me to the door; standing in the winter sunshine, with her cotton apron pulled over her thin grey hair, her arms bare, heedless of cold, she stood begging me with her eyes for a word of cheer. "Yes, Nellie," I said, answering her unspoken plea; "he's very sick today. But you know the change may come any time now. With your good care, we can hope he'll be better again in time."

"Oh Father—Doctor", she exclaimed, "I mayn't let him go this way. There's some't a'tween us as I've never told til ye. I mayn't see him go widout speakin' til him. 'Tis thirty-four years come next May him and me haven' passed the toime o' day, and us livin' in the same house all the whoile. Still, he did me a hurt long ago. Tho' 'tis no matter now, I've never said one word til him sinst; nor he til me. Ye see Doctor he mayn't go this way. Tho' indeed I kep' a good house for him all these years, and mended and darned for him. 'Tis quare how one gets to know what's needed. If he was going ploughin' I'd know by the weather and the boots he'd have on. If he was shearing the sheep I'd know by the toime o' the year and the shears in his hand. I allus knew what he'd be doin' next day. I bought and mended his clothes for him. He allus put the money in the sugar bowl on the dresser, and I was free of it, but never a word we said, one til t'other. But he mayn't go like this, Doctor. I maun say til him I'm glad he wouldna agree to me taking Dennis Murphy, him that's dead and gone this long toime; God rest his poor wicked soul. Ye see, I was old. Dennis wanted me. His auld mother was gone, but Michael would never agree. His last words to me were, "If ye was never to speak to me again, Nellie, I don't want ye to go to the likes o' him." So we never spoke again from that day to this. But we stayed together, because there was naught else to do, now was there? He needed me, I needed him, but now that he's going I must say til him I'm glad he wouldn't let me go to Dennis Murphy. I must speak to him. Won't you help me, Doctor?"

I went back to Michael. As best I could, I made him understand, in spite of his extreme weakness, that Nellie wished to speak to him. With understanding came a look of happiness and contentment over his worn face. I knew things would be all right, and I stole out into the gathering dusk, making my way home in the soft winter twilight. Next day, a happiness reigned on the faces of Nellie and her brother. No improvement in his condition was noticeable, but a contentedness, not there before, was in his eyes. No reference was made to the night before, but it was plain to see that we had all begun to hope again.

That night, a great storm came. For three days I was kept from seeing Michael. For three days I kept wondering how he was, wondering if the change had come, wondering which change. On the fourth day, I made my way over the drifts, slowly, heavily, ploughing the last mile on snowshoes, with the bright yellow March sun overhead. The change had come. Michael was better. With the certainty of living, a change had come also in the feelings of the pair, whether from long habit, whether because disuse had wasted their ability to talk, or had made talking unnecessary, or whether another disagreement had arisen; Nellie and Michael were no longer on speaking terms. I still see them on summer days, still talk to them one by one. They are both grateful for Michael's recovery. Their lives run on as before, in silence, nor does either one refer to it. I am left wondering; after all—silence is golden.

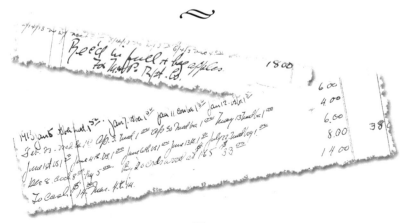

Medical Economics

THERE IS A LIGHTER SIDE to medical economics, in spite of all the ink spilt, and all the words spoken, concerning tariffs and fees and fee splitting, hours of work, partnerships, money made and lost, pensions, retirement plans and annuities. These are all heavy subjects, about which many doctors know little, and are subjects not to be taken too seriously, except by expert economists, who, in any case, never agree among themselves.

I got my introduction to this important side of medicine when I came, looking for an apprenticeship, to a typical country doctor's home. Delicious citron jam was on the table for supper that night. "Forty dollar" jam, it was called. Dr. Stevenson, my Preceptor, had worked, over the years, for a certain family living on the top of a sunny mountain, where the roads were abominable, but where citrons grew, large and juicy, while the head of the house sat in the sun, by the back door, whittling a stick. Ten children had he; "Ma wants worm powders, from Lizzy down—Maggie's bokin' and pukin' awful bad; come as soon as you can, Ma says.—Me wooman's took awful bad! De baby's comin', she dinks." Forty dollar citron jam was the net result to the doctor, that summer and for many summers, before and after.

Long ago, in the 1870s, the Presbyterian minister got, as a marriage fee, a heaped up basket of fresh blackberries. Evidently customs and ways of life were not changing very fast hereabouts. Thirty years later, Josephine, a long-time patient, very happily took her flock of Christmas turkeys to the village store. Then she came across to my office to give me a couple of turkeys, too scrawny for the store. As a bonus she brought three bantam roosters as well—with all their pretty feathers left on—"Tiens, mon cher Monsieur le Docteur, who has done so much for us."

Handling loose straw, loading and unloading it, is a formidable job. There is lots of dust, pollens, thistles and seeds. Sammy built a generous load and brought it five miles, to bed down my horses. He was a prosperous farmer; he liked money, but in the bank in his own name, even though he owed me a goodly sum. Sammy had a lot of trouble building that load and it was good clean straw. He thought that straw such as this, was worth at least thirty dollars on his doctor's account—even if the "going" price was nearer twelve. Poor Sammy was very upset when he was sent home with his full load.

With thirteen childbearing women in the village there were, each year, from nine to twelve full-time deliveries or a corresponding number of miscarriages. During the depressed thirties the grocer was owed monumental sums—the people had to live! The doctor's accounts were comparable monuments.

I needed a garage, and ordered two thousand five hundred feet of lumber. Old Joe, working in the mill, undertook to pay for it by deductions from his wages, over the indefinite future. The garage was built and the lumber merchant sent in his bill for three thousand five hundred feet. I protested, but he insisted "It is not my fault if your carter threw off part of the load before he got to your place." I had the lumber measured in the building. It was two thousand seven hundred feet, and Old Joe insisted that he had paid the bill.

The merchant accepted my cheque for the total amount. Both Joe and the merchant are long dead but Joe's bill lives on. Was the merchant twice paid? Depression economics continued to become more complicated.

Payments, if any, were made largely in kind. Our cellar filled up with bags of potatoes. There had been a good crop, those years. Spring was coming, and the cellar had to be emptied; patients were hungry and potatoes were good food. Rarely did I set out on a call without a couple of bags of potatoes in the cutter. About the same time a farmer with an old cow, for which he had no fodder, was offered three dollars and fifty cents for the whole cow, on the hoof. In normal times that would have been the price of a good cow hide. One other solution was to bring a chunk to me, on the bill. Our shed, one winter, was hung around with quarters of beef, of pork, and mutton. Again it was distributed in the cutter.

Edouard had a tuberculous mother and many children. He owed, over the years, owed considerably, but wished to pay. He owned some desirable lake-side cottage lots, of little value to him. At his request I accepted some lots on account, and a large part of his bill was wiped out. Two cottages were built to sell, and later a third one for myself.

The first two sold easily, just in time to send my first two sons to school in Ottawa. The buildings, with field stone fireplaces, were of logs, cut by local unskilled labour at one dollar per day cash and one dollar off their old accounts. In fact, some of it was in advance, for those expecting an increase in the family in the following months. Some days the builders would be fifteen in number and sometimes twice as many, when the logs, squared on two sides at the mill, were too long and heavy. Handcut cedar shingles covered the roof and fieldstone chimneys complemented the fireplace.

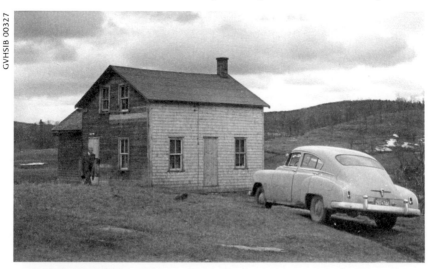

GVHSIB 00327

A remote house-call.

One fireplace smoked abominably, and had to have a new face, to bring the chimney flue into proper relation with the face, to stop the smoke nuisance. This gave it a handsome extra mantle on which to display brass, pottery, bric-a-brac, or local floral and geological specimens. In point of fact, it was this extra mantle that sold the cottage after a few months!

We still own and use the third cottage. It was an old, squared cedar log house built by early settlers, probably one hundred and twenty five years before, and one of the second crop of residences after the first primitive shanties. More recently it had been used as an open shelter, full of hay, where the farmer had let his cattle shift for themselves. With it, a smaller log building had been used as a pig sty. Truck men numbered each log, hauled them over five miles of frozen lake and farm roads to the new site, on a rocky bluff, in a clump of cedars and pines, looking right into the sunset.

The cottage was ready for occupation in a few months and cost, in cash, less than one thousand dollars! The rest was on "dead horse" accounts. The furniture, too, and much of the drapes and rugs were locally made. The wife of one poor chap, dying of cancer of the stomach, paid her account with thirty yards of home woven "Catalogne" (rag) rugs. Six birch chairs were made one winter by another man. In the spring the seats and backs were woven from the green inner bark of the standing swamp elm—all on old accounts We all survived the years of depression; many were hungry and many of the debts remain.

Poor Whites

THE MESSAGE WAS CLEAR and unmistakeable. Thirty miles separated us. Tom, with his Irish facility of speech and Irish cunning, made me feel that Mary really did have pneumonia. Sorry I was that the wires had weathered last night's storm, sorry that Tom pleaded so eloquently and persuasively for his sick wife. Still, there was no help for it, the four- or five-hour trip must be faced. Luck was with me all the same; it was not night, fresh horses, early hour, bright sunshine, wooded hills and valleys even if a muddy road. A lovely prospect for the eye to offset the fatigue of the journey, and almost certainly, as the Old Doctor would have said, "God was their Paymaster," his whimsical way of saying that they would not be able to pay for it.

But if God was their Paymaster, He must have been far away when Tom settled where he built his home. A wide level tract of some twenty acres in one piece, unusual in our world, backed by an abrupt bare rocky hill, some fifty or sixty feet high, lying like some undulating sea monster left high and dry by a receding tide. To the south east, just next to the rising sun, where the rock rose up to two hundred feet, seemed to be the monstrous head. To the south and west the plain was bounded by murmuring pines and hemlocks swaying and drooping their burdens of last night's wetness. An effective windbreak this bush made. One felt one could seek nothing further beyond its shadows.

The logs Tom cut each winter in this forest brought him ready money. Tom, with the same hatred of the bush shared with his father from their hard struggle clearing the land, shunned the shelter of the trees and built his house out in the centre of his twenty acres, where every wind that blew came near to blowing his roof off, and where the fierce rays of the July sun had full play to scorch and burn. Not a tree or shrub grew near his log house. Only the stumps remained, mute evidence of the magnificent pines that Tom's father had hated, and in his hate destroyed in years gone by.

His home stood out, one lone, bleak four-square log house, with sloping roof, crooked door, crooked window frames, crazy stove pipe chimney. At a little distance was a stable, low, log-built, with a straw stack at one end and a hay stack at the other, showing that Tom was a farmer. Two or three shaggy, mangy cows, a long-haired, long-legged, long-eared, long-nosed, lanky pig wandered about from stable to house, from house to water hole, and back again to the shelter of the stacks. To this extent Tom was a farmer. Altogether, his farm was a ruin, a castle of despair; far removed from the sheltering hills or the mysterious woods. Nothing hid its harshness and nakedness except when winter's snows covered the ugly man-made scar that it was.

Leaving the horses sheltered and blanketed by the stack, Tom, with his gallant Irish ways and speech, brought me to his home. He was tall, clean shaven (two weeks ago,) red faced, blue eyed, getting white haired I could see, where his tightly fitting red toque allowed some of his hair to show. Dressed in a ragged sweater of brown wool, and patched pants of many colours and fabrics, he carried himself like a king, unconscious of his elephantine feet, covered by huge rawhide moccasins swathed about the ankles with numerous cloths and bandages.

"Yes, yer honour, yes Doctor, we've been living here many's the year. I was born'd here. I came back from Ioway sixteen years ago when I was married, to look til the aud folks." Then he resumed: "She's very sick, been coughin' and ailin' these five weeks she has, but never left her work 'til two days agone, yer honour. Can't eat nothink, your reverence, excuse me, yer honour, so what she can't; she's got that bad a taste 'til her vittles."

And so, on and on, until, having left off my coat, I made for the stairway, picking my way between the chairs, the table, the stove, the dogs, the children, blue-eyed and pretty, the four or five sets of footwear spread out to dry on the floor near the stove, and the countless other litter that stood in my way. The floor itself was in holes, but it mattered little, for it rested directly on the earth beneath; where the boards failed, the earth was there to take its place. Not so the stairway; creaky, ladder like, old and worn. I tripped and barked my shins, and in another moment, straightening up, I bumped my head on the floor above.

At last I was beside Tom's Mary. Thirty miles I had come, and at a glance, no pneumonia, but a very much worn out, almost white-haired old woman of forty-two. Wracked with neuralgia, torn by coughing, poisoned by sixteen of the most vile tooth stumps one could imagine. Mary sat up in bed and bewailed her fate. Seven children she had; three pretty little girls, eight, seven and five years of age. An older one of fifteen had lost her prettiness in facing the stern realities of life. There were three boys; the oldest sixteen; not a trace of childish prettiness about them—already mature, though small, shrunken and unpromising. However, Annie would get me some dinner. "Sure, after coming so far, ye can't go without something. Annie'll get the meat ready. The tea's been waiting ready this last hour; it'll be good now; just sit in and make out y'r dinner."

There was no lack of kindness, but total lack of the appreciation of the amenities, or crudities of life. In spite of my protests, in spite of my best stories about it being my fast day: "a Presbyterian fast is very severe; you can't eat anything at all, all day." In spite of my pocket lunch eaten just before I arrived; in spite of my chronic stomach requiring carefully spaced meals; in spite of stories that had satisfied many a French household, hospitality was not to be escaped in this home. A sheet was spread on the rickety table, leaning against the wall. Bread, heavy and sour, butter with crystals of salt glistening on its greasy surface, brown sugar in a bowl well stained with the marks of many a dipped spoon, and mould-topped preserved blueberries were laid on the table.

A three legged backless chair was placed in front of a knife, fork and spoon, and a much-chipped stoneware cup and saucer. The meat was almost ready, "freshening" in the pan. Soon the water would be poured off; the frying or hardening process would begin.

Minute after minute preparations went on, while I pulled Mary's teeth; trying all the time to beat them to it, and escape the fully prepared meal. But her teeth were a tough proposition, and though I am proof against anything medical, a filthy, bloody, stinking mouth is hardly a good preparation for a meal. Finally, I was done; and Mary lay waking a bit from her chloroform, half angry at me, although glad at the same time that her mouth was free of teeth and would have a chance to heal up. Done, too, was the meat in the pan. What to do about it was the next question. On another occasion, I would have downed some of the stuff, thanked them heartily and made off; but this time, with visions of Mary in the loft above, I simply could not eat; could not, even if life itself depended on it. In any case, I thought, I need not mind offending them. They'll never be able to give me a cent for my trouble; "God is their Paymaster." So, packing up and getting into my coat, to the chorus of protests from the family, I made for the door. But I had not noticed Tom; there he stood, money in hand. God was not their Paymaster after all. Tom paid his bill. I had offended him by not eating in his home. He'd not call me again— thank goodness.

The Years Between III

TYPHOID FEVER WAS ALWAYS on our minds in the early days; the wonder is that it is not with us still, for our sanitary conditions are not as different even yet. If a temperature had kept up for a week; if the patient had had a nose bleed; if he'd not taken to his bed at once; if he had headache and loss of appetite, then look out for typhoid fever. Institute bedside antiseptic measures and use typhoid para-typhoid vaccines on the whole household. If the vaccine did no good, it at least kept visitors away, for it became my habit to inoculate any visitor who happened to be found in contact, willing or not. There was one case that got me great credit, for his suggestive symptoms cleared up as by a miracle within a week. His grandmother gave the credit to the few tablets of quinine I had given him for the headache. This was before the days of household aspirin. It used to be said that he who knew typhoid, knew medicine. Osler's "The Practice of Medicine," edition 1911, had some eighty pages on typhoid, its course, its complications, and its nursing.

Today's medical textbooks have a scant page on the subject. Yet we had epidemics such as the Gelinas family, eighteen miles from the railway station. Few visitors they'd had that hot summer, when I was called to see "grandmère" with a temperature of 105 degrees Fahrenheit. Ill for three weeks, she was dead in a few days. All the family crowded in. One wee grandson was lying on the floor of an empty room, trying to put up with a high temperature. He died too, very soon. By Christmas time, there had been twenty-six cases, all Gelinas, two deaths at home and eleven deaths in hospital during the second and third week of the illness. Of one family, the mother and eight children died, two remained; one of them a deaf mute boy.

Then there were the Daniels, who kept a store in the village. An orphan boy returned from a lumber shanty recovering from "la grippe"; languid, great loss of weight and no strength. In three weeks seven Daniels were ill, father and mother and all five children. "La Thom" was their Florence Nightingale, giving them baths, doing the washing, changing the beds, disinfecting clothing and disposing of excreta week after week. "La Thom" deserved well of her neighbours, though she was very much of an outcast herself; "a sage femme" and part-time abortionist. "La Thom" would undertake anything; she made up for her easy-going lazy husband, doing bush work or shingling the barn as needed. Her heart eventually failed. She had a long disheartening decline, and there was no nurse for her in her time of need. She deserved well of her people.

La Chute had an epidemic of typhoid fever. The parson's wife took ill. No diagnosis was made, no anti-typhoid precautions were taken. The whole family crowded in to visit. Within a month I was called twenty-six miles towards La Chute in the last week of November, across our hardly frozen river. Separating the team of horses, we led them across one by one, and went back to pull over the cutter, harnessing up the team on the far bank. It grew warm that November day, and rain began to fall. When I got back after dark, the river was no longer frozen. I crossed in a boat. My horses remained on the far bank until, by Christmas week, the ice was again strong enough for a safe crossing. Nevertheless, my horses had a busy month, with three or four trips each week, to ever another victim of a severe type of typhoid.

One young woman died in February, infected by the meddling of her troublesome old mother, who had no use for antiseptic measures. My last trip to that epidemic was in the last days of March of the next year. I had had a good training in the complications of typhoid fever.

Then there was the old village blacksmith. Two consultants saw him, but decided he was only "an old man going out with chronic nephritis". Five of his family contracted typhoid in the fourth week of his illness, about the time his Widal test at last proved positive. The disease then jumped several houses up the road, and three cases developed; one old lady died, the other two, a young child and her oldish father, were seriously ill with many complications for three long winter months. The only contact was the village well, which is still in use today.

The Redemptorist Fathers had a summer monastery on one of our lakes. Madame Ernest, on the neighbouring farm, had a good market feeding the seventy-five students for the long summer holiday, milk, cream and butter. Two cases of typhoid had occurred in Madame Ernest's family, but Madame herself had not been ill. It also developed among the students and they were evacuated to hospital, where one died. All the rest went home. The next year, the same thing happened; also the next year again. Early the following spring, two of the farm girls had typhoid and recovered. No students took ill. The next year Ernest took ill, with severe bowel haemorrhage and died of exhaustion after many weeks. Then Madame Ernest herself had typhoid fever and recovered. That year also, a severe outbreak of the fever occurred at the monastery.

The next spring I was asked to inoculate the whole group on their arrival at the lake. Taking a 20 cc syringe with an alcohol flame to disinfect the needle, I jabbed the whole group. When halfway through, I noticed that I had given a double dose to each victim. I was not a popular visitor the next week, when it came time for the second dose, but I assured them the reaction would not be so severe this time.

Finally, a newly appointed county health nurse managed to prevail on Madame Ernest's family to cooperate. In making examinations, Madame Ernest herself was the carrier, and could no longer sell to the Redemptorists.

A power company built three huge dams on our river. Several thousand labourers came together. They drank untreated river water, and lived in barracks or improper shacks. Dysentery developed; a few went to hospital, some died; most of them were allowed to go to their homes, where typhoid fever was diagnosed. How many in this epidemic there were, no one ever knew. Most got little or no attention. No one ever knew how far the infection spread by men going to their homes. I had the experience of two small outbreaks. The company began to treat the water, and the epidemic died out. A second corporation, in 1941, started to build a plant and quarry, and again a large group of men assembled. River water was again in use on a large scale. Typhoid vaccine was administered to all who would take it. It is probable that almost every man got one or more doses, but in any case, no typhoid developed.

Over the years, scarlet fever has lessened very much in severity. Not many years before my arrival, an epidemic of scarlet fever wiped out the whole of one family, eight or nine children, in the space of a few weeks. There were such severe throats with scarlet fever that we always gave large doses of anti-diphtheria serum, in case we might be dealing with a double infection. I feared scarlet fever for myself for some reason, but not diphtheria. I remember well one bright winter day, going far back to the end of a bush road to a mother with a child dying of scarlet fever and acute nephritis. I stayed with her that afternoon, as she was in quarantine, and no neighbour could or would come to her. Her husband was away in the bush, and I stayed until the child died in convulsions.

In 1915, I had an outbreak of scarlet fever four miles from home. Several cases were mild and untreated but one boy developed gland infections in his neck, needing incisions. By then also, he had developed acute nephritis. The mother would not listen: "The others got better without you; he will too." He got better in 1915, to die in 1957 of chronic nephritis, leaving a wife and four children, after several years of heroic modern treatment.

In 1916, a girl recovering from a family-wide epidemic of scarlet fever, developed nephritis, and some days later, pneumonia, which was followed by empyema (lung abscess). Doctor Pritchard and I drove eighteen miles one bright winter day and removed a rib in her home, as she would not be accepted in a hospital. She died several weeks later. The advent of sulpha and antibiotics, particularly penicillin, since World War II, has changed scarlet fever, and has almost eliminated the serious late complications of heart disease and kidney disease. Even with these "wonder drugs" scarlet fever is still to be feared.

A widespread disease was goitre in all its manifestations. In school, when on smallpox vaccination visits, it was quite usual to find six or eight of the ten children with a smooth or nodular enlarged neck. It was noticeable how it affected certain families. There were three such families in the Wolf Lake region, the members of which were nearly all goiterous. Someone has said that goitre causes sterility, but this was never a feature there. The neck enlarged during pregnancy, and often retracted after the baby came. When Lugol's iodine solution was used, the neck would not enlarge in the same way, and not so often had we newborn babies with big nodular thyroids. Thyroid extract or iodine became routine in all pregnancies.

There were originally many cases of enormous goitres, people in their sixties and seventies, with more or less inactive thyroids. Yet, in going into the history, a woman would admit having periods of undoubted toxic symptoms, with or without pregnancies. At times fit for much hard work, they were at other times too fatigued, too weak and too nervous to accomplish anything. Some of these became permanently hyperthyroid, and the circulation suffered. A number of these, as a result of surgery, got great benefit, and lived on into old age. Some middle-aged women, menopausal or younger, became violently ill with almost uncountable pulse rates, great loss of weight, big appetite and the inability to rest or sleep. They had small nodular goitres, "irritable heart" they were called by my Preceptor, and he treated them over the months by bed rest, sedation, and Ammonium Chloride with Tincture of Iodine locally to the neck. Some recovered and some remained ill for years. "Poison her with iodine," I was advised by a consultant one Thanksgiving day, when, after a round trip of some forty-five miles, and seeing seventy-two "big necks", we saw this acute toxic goitre. I did as he said. She blessed me for her itchy rash and scaling, but she lived for years in comparative freedom from thyroid intoxication. While toxic symptoms flowed or ebbed, the greatly enlarged necks did not change much in size or texture. A patient at Duclos, I used to think of in connection with the old trade sign of the pawn broker. On the right, such a mass, that the head was tilted to the left to allow the mass to fit between the lower jaw and the collar-bone. On the left, it was almost as large, and the central area was as large as a medium sized grapefruit.

Then, the mother of one family, who had "le coup plein" as it was euphemistically called, carried under her blouse a large pendulous mass attached to her neck by a very small stalk, and hanging down as low as her breasts. In profile, she could hold the thyroid mass at right angles to her neck with her flexed arm. Yet, toxic symptoms were for the most part absent or not noticeable. This woman lived a long hard life and died after years of cardiac failure. All her daughters had big necks and big families. There were several brothers, all with huge necks, developed, they considered, from being the bottom man on the saw in the old fashioned sawing pit. They were all sub toxic or mildly toxic. In each case the circulation failed, and they died of cardiac failure. Operation then was not considered, nor was "grosse gorge" considered a disease.

Mrs. L was another with a huge family of sixteen or seventeen; carrying each one brought such a change in size and hardness of her goitre that her respiration was greatly disturbed. She became maniacal, finally died of circulatory failure, permanently insane, leaving daughters with big necks, and big psychiatric problems. Another lady could be heard breathing half way across the yard, as she carried two pails of milk to the house. When she developed pneumonia, her fate was sealed. She died in less than thirty-six hours.

With the coming of iodized salt for animals and man, the goitre picture has totally changed. Now and again we find an active thyroid; seldom do we see goitre in schools, and operations are few and far between. Tuberculosis was ever present; not the old chronic patient who has survived many years, such as we meet today, but the active type that wiped out family after family, seemingly without any prospect of cure. One after another, over a period of some ten years, six or seven of one family died. The whole of another family of eight also died in about ten years; and of a third family, only two who had left home before the disease began, remained alive after eight or nine years. The father had come to me for something for one of the first girls to die, and I took the opportunity to say; "Can you not have all your household X-rayed and examined, and try to save some of them?" Smiling, the father questioned: "Pensez vous qu'on attrape cette maladie là?—Do you think that disease is infectious?"

Within a year he himself had a pain in his neck; a wisdom tooth was removed but the pain persisted. I was called one morning; he was paralysed from the neck down, his head crooked over to one side. A halter to extend his neck fracture, and a suprapubic catheter, gave him comparative relief for his last three weeks. His remaining son, who missed the infection, today has a "TB complex", but he has no disease.

The tuberculosis phobia engendered in certain families has lasted three or more generations, most of the second generation having died of it. The third refuses to be X-rayed or even to go to a doctor for fear of being told the truth. The doctor was often anxious not to let the patient know he was suspecting it, or even looking for it. Once suspicion was aroused, doctor number one

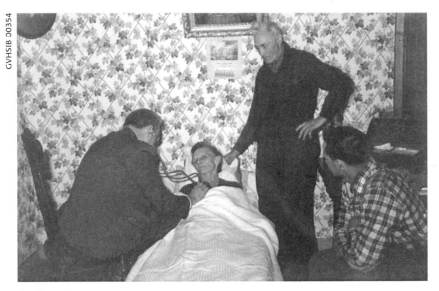

GVHSIB 00354

Anxious times.

would lose the patient and doctor number two, who was perhaps more cute or more lucky, would take over. "This man gives me hope; you gave me none," said a father when changing doctors for his son with acute miliary tuberculosis, who of course died a few weeks later. He had been ill some six months, losing weight, coughing and spitting while he worked in a city dairy.

We had our bone cases and our cervical gland cases but they were rare. Bovine TB has not been a great question among us, perhaps because our cattle do not stand in stables all winter. With the increase in knowledge; with the isolation of open cases in free sanitaria beds; with the early X-ray diagnosis of cases by free travelling clinics, tuberculosis has changed. A few chronic closed cases remain with us; even these are rare after fifty years. Yet we have to keep our eyes open; it could happen again.

One bright winter Monday morning, Jason was rolling the roads after the overnight snowfall. "Will you stop in and see my missus? She has some queer spots on her face, not sick, but as you're going by, stop in and see her, please." His "missus" was baking cookies when I saw her. She'd got up early and finished the washing and hung it on the line, and now she was baking. Her Sunday visitors had eaten up all her cookies. Her three-month-old boy was in his cradle. The fifteen-month-old boy was toddling from chair to chair. The grandfather was doing the stable chores, the grandmother was patching a quilt as she rocked the cradle. It was a comfortable, rather upper-class farm home.

Mrs. Jason had seven smallpox pustules on her face. She'd had a "go of grippe" a few days before, with such a sore back. "I could not get up for three days. Then the rash came, but I'm all right now." I had vaccine in my bag, not too fresh, but at once I vaccinated the children. The grandparents had had smallpox years previously, when everyone had it. The next day, with fresh vaccine, I again vaccinated the children.

Wednesday morning I was called; the fifteen-month-old was very ill. Examination revealed nothing definite; severe infection possibly or pneumonia. Friday morning, very early, a purpuric spot like a bruise appeared on his right ankle, and that settled the question. He died that afternoon. It was purpuric smallpox, or black smallpox, or the black death of medieval times. His vaccination did not take; the baby's was successful. The grandparents blamed the doctor—"He didn't know what was the matter." By that time I'd had more experience with several small outbreaks of smallpox.

Old Jean Paul came in with a very sore back. He too had had the grippe. He said, "At least it's not smallpox", and I agreed. A few days later, I was driving up country, and there was Jean Paul buying meat from the butcher along the roadside. He was covered with early smallpox. I'd learned my lesson, and made no more mistakes. Luc and his sister Hélène were very dull children of half-witted parents. When I was called, there was hardly a two-square-inch area on either child without great pustules, like hard green peas. Their scalps were covered with pustules, and very painful. Their hair had to be cut, and puss dripped from the scissors as I cut it. The mother was angry when I put the hair in the stove; she had wanted to keep the girl's hair to make a pad for the pompadours then in vogue. The table oilcloth on the bed, propped up along the sides with pillows, made a good bath for the children; covered lightly with a flannelette sheet, they were frequently sprinkled with a watering can of warm boracic solution for the next week. Both recovered with little scarring.

It was because of smallpox that I met my artist friend. She was keeping house for her old father in her country cottage, and spent her spare time making sketches of the beauty spots among the hills and lakes of the surrounding country. An accomplished draftswoman, a sometimes too enthusiastic colourist, like the rest of us, she often hit a middle point, where draftsmanship and colour combined to make an arresting picture. Norma had been to visit her sister in the city. Her nephew had had "chicken" pox and she had sat on his bed ten days previously. Now she was liberally sprinkled with smallpox in an advanced stage, with one large confluent patch on her left cheek. She had had the usual few days "grippe" and a very sore back. The pustules around her eyes, in her scalp and on her cheek, were very painful. Even though out of sorts, she'd had a group of young skiers up from the city the weekend before, and they had returned to their various city callings, eight public schools and collegiates, and four or five business offices. There was some scrambling and hurrying in the city health department that Friday afternoon, when news reached the offices. Norma recovered, but carried a deep wide scar on her cheek for the rest of her life.

Fifteen cases of smallpox in as many years, ten small outbreaks, with three deaths; twenty per cent death rate. The old death rates were usually over thirty per cent. In one of my old medical books is written: "The disease spread like fire through the unprotected population, and there died that winter, in Montreal alone, three thousand one hundred and forty people, of which two thousand one hundred and seventeen were children under seven years of age. It took a catastrophe to open the eyes of the people to the real value of vaccination. Since that time, vaccination is carried out throughout the Province of Quebec without any opposition, with the result that that Province is freer of smallpox than any other." Ref. *Four Centuries of Medical History of Canada,* 1928. (Ed. note: *Today smallpox has been eliminated from the world by vaccination.*)

Old Bill had mined gold all over the north, and retired to boast of his hardships. His sister, Margaret, had kept house for a city public health doctor, and had come home to keep house for him. Bill had "grippe and a sore back; would I see him? He has a queer rash." He had smallpox a week old, with an early pustule in his eye. "My doctor says I can't take vaccination," was her protest when I insisted on vaccination for her. The next week, Margaret had a fully developed smallpox, and was a sorry old woman. Both recovered, but Bill had a blind eye.

Winter had just come, hard autumn roads on wheels had given place to the comfort of cutter driving, but the wind was cold where the bush gave way to level farmland. "Go in and get warmed up," I said to my six-year-old son when we got to Patrick's house, fifteen miles from home: "Go in while I blanket the horses." When I got in myself, my son was warming his hands by the stove, talking to Patrick, and eating a cake. Patrick was in an advanced stage of smallpox, with many confluent areas on his pressure points, waist band, wrists, palms, and the soles of his feet. We had been vaccinated, but my second son was only vaccinated when we got home that night. Maynard was a good friend; when he came to the office at breakfast time six years later, I picked up my third son to show the baby to my friend.

Maynard had typical smallpox. Before doing anything for him, I vaccinated my son. As I did, he jerked his arm, so he now has a crescent shaped scar on his arm. Mary and her friend were coming to the country for a summer holiday. Her friend had "grip" and could not come, so Judy went to say goodbye to her. Three days later, the news came that the friend had smallpox. I vaccinated Mary at the end of the week and it was taking nicely, but not in time to save her from a mild case with typical generalised rash. It was a lively disease; kept one guessing and alert.

Mrs. Jim was expecting her third baby that spring. She was a good butter-maker, and had many customers in the city. They had to be satisfied, even if in two months the new baby would make her "lie up" for a few weeks. To keep the butter right she would start out at three o'clock in the cool of the morning. Coming home from my frequent calls, I would meet her on the road going off to market; butter, cream, lamb and pork in the express wagon, and again in the hot afternoon, driving home with empty boxes and drooping with fatigue, the horses barely wandering along. A week later Mrs. Jim had the usual "grip" and a sore back. She, too, developed a smallpox rash that went through its four stages; within a month she had lost her baby. He was born with pustules well on to the healing stage. Mme Arthur had a large family, fifteen or more. She was expecting another baby one very cold January, twenty-six miles away. She'd had "la grippe" and the inevitable sore back; a woman having a seventeenth baby has a sore back in any case, but she developed a rash. Ten days later, with healing smallpox, she gave birth to a living baby with healing smallpox. An incubator for the four-week premature baby was set up with hot water bottles and plenty of cotton wool. The next day, when I returned, my baby was hideously scalded with too hot bottles and insufficient cotton wool. Smallpox causes premature labour.

Over the years the country doctor is judged to a large extent by his ability with his obstetrical patients. If he has any luck he is mentioned as a "specialist", even if, as in my own case, he is only too conscious of his shortcomings. I delivered sixteen maternity cases in my first six weeks, on an average of one hundred and thirty cases each year, until my son, in 1945, took over about half of them. The record year, about 1936, was one hundred and forty-four cases. In all the years, it is safe to estimate that I have attended about four thousand six hundred and sixty-four cases. One woman I delivered fourteen times in twenty-one years; her last baby had been dead for some days with a tight knot in the cord. Eight times she had a retained placenta that I had to remove manually with much haemorrhage; once she had severe phlebitis in the veins of her leg, twice she needed and got blood transfusions, all in her own home. Some women are indestructible; "Enfin le Bon Dieu est bon," was all she said about it recently when she came to see me in bed with a heart attack. It would be consoling if, as newspaper writers often say in obituaries for this or that doctor, "he attended one thousand five hundred maternity cases and never lost a

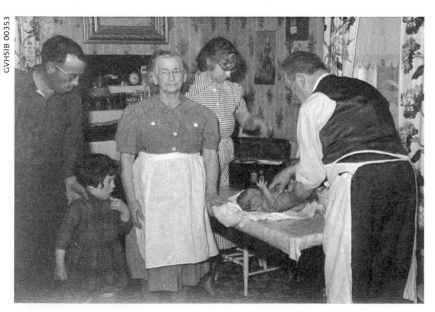

GVHSIB 00353

A healthy home delivery.

mother." I can't say that, since I must admit I lost an average of one mother every second year, perhaps one in two hundred and sixty. Since our small hospital opened in 1952, in over two thousand cases, we've lost but one mother. That was an eclamptic who collapsed on the doorstep and died, and a postmortem caesarean section saved her baby girl.

I've lost about twenty mothers over a period of fifty years, some of them preventable had adequate prenatal care been available. Under the circumstances, this was impossible; this result must be accepted. There might have been twice as many. The maternal deaths were mostly from accidental haemorrhage, a few from toxaemia, though there were many toxic cases, fewer still from sepsis or puerperal fever. Every one was an exhausted woman, exhausted from farm work, home work, too many pregnancies too close together. Some were complicated by tuberculosis, or cancer, or heart disease. Until we can have adequate birth control methods, in spite of admitted drawbacks, it is my belief that maternal mortality cannot be reduced to the ultimate minimum desirable.

I have no figures on the abortion rate; how many, or with what results. All along, there have been, within easy reach, doctors or others who for a price in advance would induce an abortion. In the early days I used to try to find out, if possible, the cause of the inevitable abortion, but after too many revelations of an unfortunate nature, I found that it was wise to "neglect" to know too much about the cause of the trouble. Of the many abortions we meet, at least a proportion are most certainly induced by someone. In spite of a rigid code, several times I got the reputation of being an abortionist: "You helped Madame X, you can help me; money is no object."

One night I spent watching with a very religious woman and her equally religious husband, as she insisted that she was aborting. There was no evidence of it except her statements. The next day I told her she was putting up a story. They left the village soon after. A year later, the husband wrote: "If I were not a Christian, I should take action against you for trying to abort my wife. My baby boy is three months old now, and he has no sign of the injury you tried to do him." Sometimes you can't win.

In my earlier years, when I had a maternity call, I left home going over in my mind each step in the problems of a safe delivery for both mother and child. "What shall I do if I get a face presentation?" I've had only two in fifty years. "What shall I do if I have a breech?" I've had many a breech; once a boy, the seventeenth in the family, and I could not deliver the head. A forty mile trip to hospital for assistance, brought a baby of seventeen and a half pounds, twenty-six inches long, dead of course. The mother still lives after all the years, a diabetic.

On my first day in Wakefield, I went to assist Dr. Stevenson on a maternity case. The long night slowly unrolled itself, punctuated by many cups of tea brought by the friendly neighbour midwife, lifesavers to the untried beginner. Years later, one winter morning, after another delivery in the same house, when the more seasoned doctor offered to drive the midwife home for breakfast after another long night vigil, the answer was, "Oh no, I can't go yet; I have to bake my bread first. You see, I'd set the bread to rise and I couldn't let it go to waste, so I just wrapped it up and brought it with me. Now I must bake it and bring home my week's supply." In those days, no self respecting housewife would think of serving baker's bread to the men folk.

Natural Childbirth

THIS ONE WAS A REAL NATURAL CHILDBIRTH, in fact the doctor was twenty miles away when the baby was born, assisted by an untrained but experienced "sage femme". It was quite normal, except that the "sage femme" in charge had perhaps "graissé le passage" to make the baby slip out more easily. The mother had had eleven or twelve already. All was well for three days, but "then someone left a window open to the April setting sun" and Mathilde got a chill. The next day she could not get up. All the local "wives tales" were adhered to; weasel skin, rognon de castor, Jack in the pulpit. Not too much light was allowed by the small window in the sick room. Relays of neighbours came to sit and watch and wait for the worsening signs; to sit and fry heavy salt pork, boil potatoes, and make tea to keep the family company. All was useless.

Mathilde continued to mutter, to have chills, to rave and talk nonsense. I was called for the first time on the tenth of May, and after a twenty-mile drive through the spring drenched, shining country, I saw that I was up against an almost insoluble problem. Interstitial saline, made on the kitchen stove, without scales, by guesswork, was administered into the flanks, and the breasts, and under the arms, left running when I departed after four hours of bathing, changing the bed, opening the window to the spring sun, making and administering eggnog, milk soup, and a cold drink of snow from the gully on the hillside, and last year's strawberry jam made by the sick woman. Once undertaken, it had to be seen through to its conclusion, with three and four trips each week needed for many weeks; not always special trips, for there were many patients to see along the route there and back. Mathilde's resistance was very low; my aseptic technique not always adequate, and infection set in. It was three weeks before she was awake to the various incisions and bi-weekly or tri-weekly painful dressings that had to be carried out. She learned to dread the doctor's coming. Meanwhile, little Mathilde was passed around among the neighbours, and well looked after. Albert the eldest, had been to school, and could read a bit, provided the doctor wrote plainly, and went over it word by word to make sure the instructions were clear. He continued, all summer, to be wakened in the middle of the night, to rub his eyes and sleepily interpret the doctor's instructions to his father. Pierre then would administer a cool drink of berry juice in linseed tea, give a cool sponge bath, turn the patient, change the bed, and do all the many things a nurse can do. It was September before the patient was able to be helped out to sit in the autumn sun and look down the road and see me coming to check up on her treatment.

Of course, this was not the only natural childbirth Mathilde had survived. She had plenty of what it takes to go through these episodes from time to time. In fact, she'd had eighteen births; one pair of twins, one unassisted placenta praevia, resulting in a dead baby and bloodless mother; but in this year of 1963, she still lives. She smiles when we meet, remembering the time she took three weeks to recognise me. She smiles; it gives her a great lift, "does something for her ego", when she sees the hospital care available to her granddaughters when their babies come. Albert kept my horses for two winters in payment for his mother's treatment. His daughter had her fifth baby in hospital the other day, not by natural childbirth, but by fully assisted birth. Albert, now sixty-two, and a grandfather seventeen times, and I, seventy-seven, met. Once more we smiled over the happenings of the summer of 1912.

WAITING by H.J.G. Geggie
The sun sinks down to the russet west;
the short day wanes.
Out over the water the swallows skim,
and back to the caves come twittering;
the day moves on, and I am waiting.
The mother struggles with her pain,
the miracle of birth to gain;
to gain! What will be the gain?
When that first faint cry is heard,
when those eyes first open on the world,
shall signs of the life to be appear?
Shall we, with far-seeing eye,
see the boy fashion, with his knife
by slow degrees, a toy;
things for which men give their lives—
pattern of the busy life to come.
Will that be the gain?
Or shall we with prophetic eye,
see the boy at school, eager the task to do,
hungrily the goal of knowledge attaining?
Back to his people coming, their priest, their prophet
and their consolation.
Will that be the gain?
Or will the babe grow into maidenhood
under the watchful mother's eye?
Lay down her play with a sigh,
take up her tasks with a song?
Be like her mother—a mother?
Bring to her home the joy of love,
the joy of suffering, the joy of fatherhood,
and, in old age, the joy of contentment,
after a life of giving?
Will that be the gain?
Or will stern fate snuff out the life unborn,
make of this labour on this waning day, a loss;
add grief to mother's pain?
Where then will be the gain?

Getting About

GREAT CHANGES IN GETTING about the country have come over the years. My Preceptor was a great lover of his horses; patients came first, horses next, himself last. There were water holes along the roads and the horses soon got to know where they were. So did Maggie, who lived on top of the hill above one waterhole. She'd see the doctor's team coming around the curve. She knew he would stop to water his horses before getting home, and she had just time enough to change her blouse and go down the hill to get a drive to the village, I giving up my place on the seat to stand on the rear axle.

Gatineau bridges were being discussed in the 1860s. Each man wanted the bridge in his own village or backyard. No one would give in, so political action was ineffective until Father Chenier somehow applied extra influence, and the covered bridge in Farrellton was built in 1914. The next year the Gendron Bridge in Wakefield was completed. There were few or no roads to get to these bridges.

In dry weather the way across the fields was possible; in wet weather at times it was necessary to unhitch the team in the middle of the field and leave the buggy, axle deep in mud, while man and horses staggered to safety. Gradually, over the months and years, roads were laid out, drained and surfaced to an adequate degree, and we began to enjoy our bridges, and go many a mile around to cross on them instead of on the old scows.

These scows were the only way to get across the river for many years. Many were maintained at public expense and at considerable cost. They were about fifteen feet wide by twenty feet long, with sides some two feet high and a railing of another foot or so. Back and front were brought up so as to take the water more easily, and also provide a gangway for the horses and vehicles to get on and off. Fifteen-to-eighteen-foot oars were balanced as to be not too heavy for even one man to be able to manage. At some places, scows took advantage of the river currents, with an adjustable wing balanced about the middle of the scow so that the considerable river current could push it across the river. These were cable scows attached to a cable running across the river, and were a great luxury, once the formula was mastered. At other points, the eddies along the river banks made cable scows and wings impractical; the scow then was at the mercy of the currents and eddies, with nothing to prevent the crossing being really dangerous and being swept into the rapids below.

At the time of high spring water, in the first week of May, old Fred and I pulled our hearts out, spent three hours crossing the river at Copeland's landing, time and again missing the eddy at the far side. We drifted far down within a mile of the rushing waters over the Cascades. Only by catching an overhanging branch were we able, at last, to land two miles below the regular spot.

One great difficulty with scows was the floating logs. The cable scow could be stalled in mid river with dozens and dozens of logs piled up against it. The free scow could be made unmanageable, and the man and team become helpless in the currents. Often enough, men along the banks would have to row out in boats to the rescue. Even though the horses were invariably well behaved, the prospect at night, when alone and tired, was anything but enviable, especially if the wind was up the river, slowing the logs. In November, in the first days of early frosts, scows, gathering layer upon layer of ice, became very heavy and unwieldy. Then they were hauled up on the bank until spring.

Sometimes one could use the train. There were two or three trains a day to Maniwaki, and return.

A short time before Dr. Stevenson died, we had a talk about buying a motorcar, but we came to the conclusion these contraptions would never be useful in our work! Horses were more reliable. Four years later, in 1915, I bought my first Ford for

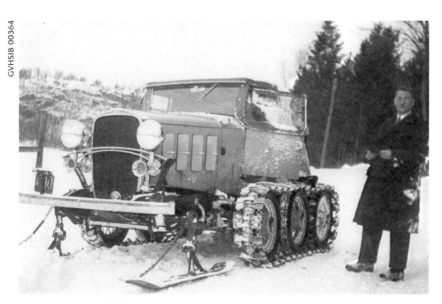

GVHSIB 00364

First snomobile. 1930s.

$615 cash! Then came a Chevrolet 490; they were never very reliable, and I always said that I learned to swear driving the Ford. The 490 was so called, it is said, because it was on the road for four days, and in the garage for ninety. The fervent hope was that the crown gears in the 490 would hold out until one got home. We had no garage nearer than Ottawa and few mechanics anywhere. I had to import gasoline and oil in drums, and do most of my repairs myself. I never went out without a dozen spark plugs, and to do ten miles without trouble was rare. Of course the horse was still supreme in the fall, winter and spring. The other advantage to a horse was that it could drive itself, at least on the way home, when I could get some sleep.

Often I had five horses on pasture, a car stuck on the road, and I was trying to rent horses or a car to keep ahead of the stork. Little wonder that with the first snow I was glad to put by the car until I got a new one in the spring, and relax watching the stars and feeling the wind as I drove my horses perhaps twenty hours per day.

Part of all this trouble was the state of the roads. The snow and the clay were hard to beat, and it was only with the passage of many years that motoring became really practical.

By the late 1930s, snow machines started to be developed. First I acquired a Ford roadster that was converted for snow travel in the winter, with skis on the front, and six wheels with heavy chains on the back. That one was replaced by a similar apparatus using a Chevrolet rumble-seat sports car. In 1940, Bombardier Company had developed a machine with four skis and a Ford engine at the back, with an aeroplane-type propeller to push it along. Very successful it was also, especially on roads broken by horses and sleighs. It was not warm or comfortable nor was it very good if the snow was wet. The brake was a loop of heavy chain which was thrown over the front ski.

In the spring, trips had to be planned to take place at night or early morning when the temperature was low enough to make a firm road. Before the bridges were built ice roads were marked out on rivers and lakes as soon as they had frozen enough to walk on. Rows of evergreen branches were placed to warn the traveller not to stray off the road, where the ice was known to be safe. During the spring break up, these roads would remain safe much longer than the rest of the ice. Many horses became wise about the safety of the ice, and would warn the driver and only proceed with urging and reassurance. The Old Doctor travelled with someone to help with the horses, or if there were problems. Much of the time this was his wife or one of his children. In the hungry 1930s, I always had a chore boy to accompany me, to look after the horses or the snowmobile. Two of these boys were Ernie Brown from Rupert, and Eusèbe Meunier from Farm Point.

Bugs

Sᴛ. Jᴏsᴇᴘʜ, ᴘᴀᴛʀᴏɴ sᴀɪɴᴛ ᴏғ ᴛʜᴇ ғᴀᴍɪʟʏ, had kept us very busy. Night after night that winter, with horses, propeller-driven snowmobile, or summer car with chains on the four wheels, we tried to keep up with his demands.

At 2 a.m. on a frosty night, we had put up the snowmobile after a twenty-eight-mile drive over hard dry snow, only to take out the team at 4 a.m., because the weather had turned soft and rain threatened. We knew that the skis would clog up with half frozen snow, making progress impossible. Lying low in the shanty cutter, Eusèbe would sleep, while I, half asleep, drove, reins around my neck, hands on the lines, dreaming "would St. Joseph ever let up, let up and let us rest?"

Three-thirty in the morning, "Eusèbe, wake up; the snowmobile this time." The snow was crisp and dry. Fifteen miles was soon over, and by noon St. Joseph was satisfied with an eight-pound, ten-ounce boy. Yet a message was waiting at the crossroads when we got there. "Fred's wife was sick, needed a doctor at once." And so, eating a pocket lunch through the March sunshine, the snow ever softening, we scurried, afraid that if we hesitated the skis would clog and make it impossible to get going again. By two o'clock we were thirty-two miles away in the middle of a great sunlit expanse of softening snow, overlooking Fred's house, where his sheet-white toxic wife was awaiting her fifth baby. Eusèbe, curling up comfortably in the robes in the snowmobile, in the full heat of the March sun, promptly went to sleep, while I, carrying my bags, made my way down to Fred's house.

There was lots to fear in the case; extreme anaemia, a dreadful mouth of foul teeth, puffy face and limbs, and no prenatal care. "Gertie had always been like this. No doctor had been able to help her, so we did not call you 'til it was time." Lots to fear, but little to do at the moment, but await the effects of medication;

meanwhile, a chance to sleep. Gertie was downstairs beside the kitchen stove, but there was a bed upstairs empty, and Mrs. Jim the midwife got it ready. It was only tolerably inviting, but lack of sleep made any bed welcome, so in no time I was asleep. Three hours later, five o'clock, the sun was getting low; the snow was crisping up nicely, making our get-away more sure. Eusèbe was cold and in he came. Meanwhile Gertie was needing me, and Eusèbe took my place, and was soon asleep on the same bed.

My patient was keeping me busy. I had no time to doze; all my attention was concentrated on her. Would she convulse? Would she live? Would the baby live? Down the stairs clumped Eusèbe, and in no unmistakable French, raged, "Les maudits Irlandais sàles. Les maudits plein de poux. Ca brûle comme du feu. J'en ai partout!" In this purely English-speaking home, he was fairly safe, but I could not help wondering if Fred would not interpret his expression, his manifest rage, his scratching at his flea bites, as

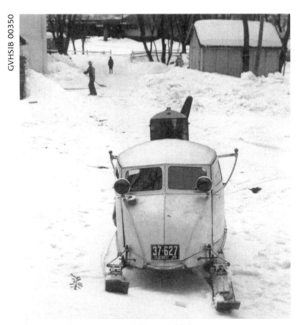

GVHSIB 00350

Bombardier snowmobile, c.1939.

he sat in a far corner, muttering and scolding half aloud. All most interesting; sunset and darkness had brought out the bugs, which I in daylight had been spared.

Midnight came, and Gertie and her miserable daughter were safe enough to leave. Supper in such a place was impossible. The snow was crisp, Eusèbe drove like one possessed with the devil of speed, muttering above the noise of the propeller. Not until we got him into an antiseptic bath was he satisfied.

St. Joseph did not relent, did not take a rest. Night after night, day after day, the pressure kept up. Ten days later we were in a French-speaking shack. It was a two-room house with a loft room above, in which there was a wide double bed and a "banc lit" against the opposite wall. Eusèbe slept in an easy chair downstairs on a sunny afternoon. Too soft this time for the snowmobile. The horses were stabled and comfortably eating, and nothing to do for the moment. I slept on the "banc lit".

About 6 a.m., light well advanced, pains getting sharp, I awoke. The sage femme was busy collecting good fat French bed bugs from my white shirt sleeves, where they showed up to better advantage than on her own dark blouse. Ever since, she has been known as "la trieuse de poux" (the Louse Gatherer). She had little else to do but pick bugs, while a new citizen made his appearance into this complicated world.

Down the stairs I went, scolding to Eusèbe in good lusty English, discussing the merits and demerits of English versus French bugs. My turn for the antiseptic bath and the clothes on the line. Eusèbe and I have never been able to agree on the question, but we do agree that bilingualism is a good way to let off steam in the face of household problems if you choose your audience well.

Keeping the Promise

IT WAS LATE MARCH at the end of a long snowy winter when one night a woman called, after driving five miles to the nearest telephone, asking me to see her husband. " 'Mède was very ill," she said, "had been a long time, in bed three months, now dreadful night sweats, pain in his chest, a bad cough, couldn't eat, vomited often. Come early tomorrow morning so as to cross the lake on the hard frozen road. The sun gets too hot later in the day. Leave your horses to rest and feed at the foot of the hill. My father will meet you with a sleigh; too much snow up here, you'll never get through to the end of the road on wheels." She had worked it all out, even to the last detail. It was only two miles to walk.

By this time I was an old hand at meeting trouble. I started on the crusty frozen mud before the sun rose, to make the best of conditions. No longer "le jeune docteur", now "le petit docteur sans chapeau" drove the horses, for I never wore a hat and people wondered why. One by one the tiny night lights shining dimly through windows, were replaced by bigger lamps as the women got up and began to prepare breakfast. At many a farm a smoky lantern swung from the man's hand as he made his way to the stable to look at his new calves and lambs; to feed his cows; to get ready for breakfast and harness up to go for the last load of logs across the frozen creeks and swamps, before the rising sun would make it impossible.

More than one person, making his way to the stable, waved a hand as the doctor's team passed. "True, 'le petit docteur' was doing the work, but he was not like 'le vieux'. His place will never be taken." The road was not easy. Many a mud hole, thinly frozen over, gave a false sense of security. Poorly tracked out snowdrifts added variety to the way. At many a spot the track left the summer road to avoid the heavy drifts caught by the cedar fences and led across muddy stubble. Sleep might be possible in the buggy even

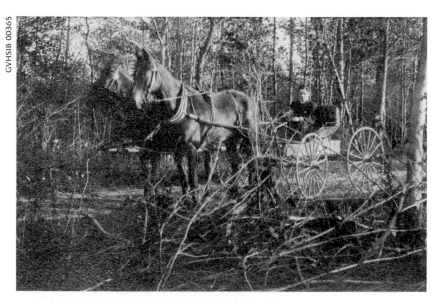

Bill Stevenson with his father's express. 1910.

on these roads on the way home, but not now, when the horses felt they were headed into the hills away from home. Mud flying, water splashing, horses plunging through mud, water and snowdrifts, one had to be alert. Yet at the end of the day, tired horses, tired man, heading home, sleep would be possible.

Slowly the sun rose. Lamps out in the homes; here and there a team started for the bush. Twenty miles gone, and another few yet to go. Then the waiting sleigh and the bustle of stabling and feeding the horses and starting off up the hill. On the big flat sleigh, with the slow-moving heavy team, there was time to dream and talk. Lots of snow up on top, yet here and there the runners cut down through it to the rock beneath, making a shuddering screechy noise as we went.

"Yes, 'Mède has been sick a long time, in fact for years, like his father. It's my idea he'll not make old bones, not that one." Slowly Baptiste told me, puffing his eternal pipe: "You remember Marie Ange said she'd marry Amède and look after him, and she did. She has four children now and has lost three. God knew she could not look after seven, so He took three." We reached the familiar clearing on the lakeshore, the same familiar stable. There was open water all around the edge of the lake, where the shore ice, frozen to the bottom, could not rise with the spring water, and it came over to cover it.

Baptiste had thrown a couple of planks across the open water, it remained only to step across onto the solid frozen winter road, and to walk two miles across the lake with my pockets stuffed with necessary drugs and equipment. The sun had risen an hour earlier, and already puddles of water were melting on the sides of the frozen road. Just beyond the roadway, the softer untramped ice was melting nicely. Here and there, there were rivulets of water pouring down through the ice, making spring music in our ears as we went. A crow, and then another crow, flapped across the icy expanse; sparrows feeding in the roadway flew to safety. At one point, as we skirted an island, a forty-foot cliff rose up, glistening in the sun, with its wetness and its icy masses. A wonderful spring morning, melting and sparkling in the sunshine, made the two-mile walk a memory.

We approached the far shore, where Marie Ange had also thrown planks across the gap of open water; but in this, for once, she had not done well enough. Perhaps the sun was too hot, perhaps I was too heavy, perhaps I stepped aside, but within a yard of the planks, down I went through the ice into the cold water and sticky mud beneath, right up to my neck! "Mon Dieu, mon Dieu," exclaimed Baptiste, already on the planks, and throwing himself down full length, he grabbed me by the hair. It was just a mischance, not a disaster, and in a moment I was on shore making my way to the shack, up the sunny slope, laughing at my predicament, but not a bit enjoying the wetting.

Marie Ange was waiting for me in the doorway with every sign of dithers on her expressive face. "What a thing to happen. I should have put out more planks, but I thought that there were enough. You'll have to put on 'Mède's suit while yours dries, you can't go home that way." Soon I was in the borrowed suit, sharing a cup of tea with 'Mède as I sat by his bedside; at least, I drank mine, while he pretended to drink his. He was very ill indeed. Between coughs he told me how he'd caught cold in the late fall when he was clearing land.

"Vous savez que a va bien, faire de la terre. I like to make land. It's cold in November, but when you get a good fire going there's nothing that smells better than the smoke. You get a protected spot and dinner seems all the better out there away from home. On est bien dans le bois. Somehow last fall the smoke did not suit me; I began coughing, and haven't been able to stop since; been in bed for three months now." A very elementary examination showed that his left chest was full up to the collar bone with fluid; his heart displaced; a right lung had a cavity in the apex; a fast pulse; and a fever of one hundred and two. Never again would 'Mède "make the land." It was tuberculosis.

While my suit dried I did a chest puncture and drew off a large bowl of bloody fluid. Slowly his heart would swing into more normal position, respiration would be easier, cough less troublesome, and fever perhaps would become less for a while. Increased comfort and sedatives might make his course easier, might give a boost to his spirits; after all, spring was coming. He could look forward to getting out in his garden, though it was pretty certain that before mid-summer it would be all over for him.

Afternoon was well on before my clothes were dry enough to change over to them, and 'Mède had a bit of a sleep. The young boys and their mother, with Baptiste, had repaired and improved the bridges on the ice. It was time to go. I walked off into the sunset along the shadowed island cliff, back to the waiting horses, thinking many things. Marie Ange was keeping the promise she had made that stormy night at the beginning of my practice, when her brother was dying.

The Telephone

ONE OF MY FIRST DRIVES WITH Dr. Hans Stevenson was to Isaie Brazeau's house on telephone business. They had, together, organised a rural party, single-wire telephone system from Wakefield to Wolf Lake and East Aldfield in Pontiac County, in 1906. The line was thirty-five miles long. M.Brazeau did much of the installation, and the doctor provided the money, his own; and from his friends, contributions of poles and labour. The exchange was at Isaie Brazeau's house in Ste-Cécile-de-Masham; later it moved a mile or so away to Norbert Martineau's place. He had been a life-long sufferer of asthma, slept very badly, and so was the best night operator available.

After some years, during the First World War, the line was pushed across "no man's land" to Quyon, through the Onslow country. By now the lines had become metallic, as hydro had come in and made the grounded lines too noisy. When I came to Wakefield, the line to Farm Point was just being built, and the switch was located, for want of a better place, in Dr. Stevenson's house. The lines were organised to facilitate the doctor's business; he had put in some $1,000 in money, and many hours of organisation and worry, to save himself many a long trip with his horses. With a party line, everyone along the road would know where the doctor was going, and, if another call came, it was often possible, by means of the phone, to locate him

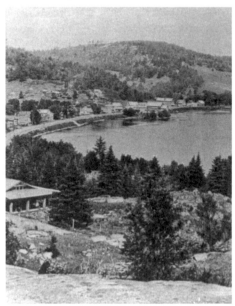

View of Wakefield looking north.

and head him off on his way home. Possible, too, for Mrs. Stevenson or a kind friend to take a fresh team to meet him at the crossroads, and bring home the tired one.

It was quite easy to ring the doctor's one long ring on a party line, and, within a few minutes, have half-a-dozen listeners, one of whom was sure to know something of the doctor's movements, and one of whom was always good enough to drive out to head him off with the message.

Somewhere in the 1920s, the switchboard was brought down to Wakefield from Norbert Martineau's, and located at Fred Wills'. There was then no night service, as the switchboard was in another building adjoining his home. Mrs. Wills was bilingual and knew everyone, and was most helpful to everyone in perplexity. For many years she did a splendid job.

After the death of Dr. Stevenson, I, as his successor in the practice, was obliged to look after the interests of the telephone company. My objective was to get at least a free exchange of messages between the four companies that radiated from Wakefield. The local authorities of each line were jealous of each other. Most of us had at least two phone boxes on our wall, but as there were four points to the compass, I had four boxes. Never did these four local lines fully exchange messages. They were: the Wakefield and Masham Telephone Company; the Rupert and North Wakefield Telephone Company, sponsored by Dr. James Pritchard and his friends; the East Wakefield Telephone Company, sponsored by Dr. Stevenson, Vital Deziel of Ste-Pierre-de-Wakefield and the progressive merchants of Poltimore, Dan McCallum and John Bonsall. The Rev. Father Ethier of East Wakefield had much to do in helping the growth of this line, and Isaie Brazeau engineered its building.

Late in the First War, Rev. Father Chenier of Farrellton interested his parishioners in building the Farrellton Rural Telephone Company. The Hydro installations were giving great troubles with the one wire grounded systems, and Father Chenier, in 1918 to 1920, built a metallic line which gave much better service than the community had before.

John Reid, manager of the Alexander MacLaren firm in Wakefield, was interested in the first three lines mentioned, for the better prosecution of the extensive MacLaren interests. In the MacLaren office there were three local telephone boxes on the wall, and also a Bell telephone. Messages could be repeated by the clerks from one system to the other, but there was no direct connection between them.

In 1911, the Bell Telephone terminal was at Dr. Kennedy's, the veterinary surgeon, next door to Dr. Stevenson in Wakefield. Calls received by Mrs. Kennedy on the Bell line, were completed only by her contacting the person on a local line, and asking them to come to the Bell office. The Bell station at Dr. Kennedy's was also the terminal of the Maniwaki Telephone line, which went on another eighty miles to the head of civilization on the Gatineau.

Perhaps the best remembered of the switchboard operators at Wakefield, was Jim Robb, who took it up when Mrs. Wills left. He was a victim of vascular disease in his legs, and after repeated surgeries, he sat for years, legless, in his wheelchair, answering the community's calls. Night or day, Jim would get to the switch in spite of his infirmities, and was helped by his sister and brother-in-law, Mr. and Mrs. Fred Moffatt.

The story is told of one lady, gossiping on the line, who happened to mention that she had beans in the oven. Jim Robb, thinking she was taking up too much time, sought to drive her off by exclaiming: "Mrs..., your beans are burning; I smell them." Difficult times came to Wakefield and its telephone lines. Poles in clay country have a limited usefulness. Thomas Brazeau, Isaie's son, took up the repair work, but he became unable to climb rotten poles. The rural lines created an interest for more than one local lad; and even today, still working in "line" work for the Bell

Telephone Company, are Brian Gorham, Harold Stevenson, and several others, who got their start with the Masham Telephone Company. Leslie Gorham went on to the Gatineau Power Company; good men they were too, teamed up with occasional helpers. Brian and his helper, my son Hans Geggie, changed the diaper of a customer's baby, leaving the telephone box ready for more gossip, and the baby happy and clean.

The era of rural phone business was going out; the Bell Company was ready and able to wait. When nothing was left but the charter and the right-of-way, Bell took over. A thousand dollars was paid for what was left of the system, with all the records, so that no one could come back on them with more or less fictitious claims. The big company had been there before, and would not make another mistake. However, we have had better service since, and the fact remains that Wakefield had telephone service before many important areas in Quebec. Within twenty-five years of the development of the telephone, Wakefield had service.

~

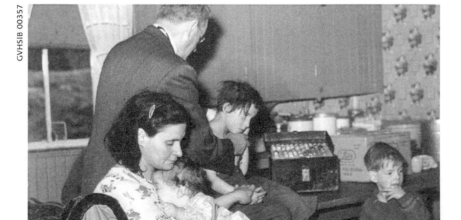

A house-call—a mother's comfort.

Popular Remedies

POPULAR REMEDIES AND MEASURES are used by my patients and midwives. Are they based on experience, on tradition, on ignorance or superstition?

There is the tradition of the "nine days." A woman has a fall or a fright, and she may expect a miscarriage in nine days. A woman has a warning or false alarm of labour, and she expects her delivery in nine days. Many will get up on the third postpartum day, and not a few will go back to bed for the famous "ninth day." Why? The old women advise it.

Then the daily taking of flax seed to "oil the passage" used to be in very common use. "Le beau mal" was a very common term. Almost any abdominal upset in a female was "beau mal". This could be all the way from gallstones with jaundice and vomiting, to cystitis and pyelitis, to extensive prolapse and bladder stones. "Rognon de castor" in gin or high wines is the remedy.

In my first years, few houses where I was called to a sick female were without a bottle of "high wine" with bits of beaver's kidney floating about in it. Many a time, my patient had an appendiceal abscess and I found her vomiting high wines with beaver kidney. It was useless for men; they did not have "beau mal". The use of roots of the wild iris for cystitis, yellow iris for men, and blue iris for women, seemed to be a relic of the ancient "mandrake". It had to be gathered at night, with special observations, to be of real value. I have seen it sold on the market at Quebec City as "Belangelique", but I have never seen it used.

In almost every expectant mother's home was an eggcup or glass of nine hand-picked grains of whole, unground wheat. Each day in the latter months, the patient would carefully count out and swallow nine grains. "J'ai pris mes neuf grains," giving surety of an easy delivery. Also "nine grains" were taken when the patient thought she was in labour. If then she thought she could lie down, she was sure that it was not time to call the doctor; and if, on the other hand, she jumped up and went to work, she knew as surely that the doctor would hardly get there in time. When I have told an expectant mother that she was not in labour, time and again a surprised look would come into her eyes and she would argue, "but I've taken my nine grains."

There is a whole host of forbidden actions. Cold water must not be given to a woman in labour. "Il faut casser l'eau" with gin or make it lukewarm. The parturant must not turn off her back or put her arms above her head, or comb her hair. She must not see a cripple or an epileptic or an unknown beggar, or dire consequences will follow, because "the old women have said so".

After the second stage of labour, after the baby is born, the cord is apt to be drawn up by a rising uterine fundus. It must be kept down, so time and again I've seen it tied to the thigh, or held by an old lady for hours, when all that was needed was to express the detached placenta. Once, after a delay of twenty-four hours, I was asked to drive twenty-six miles with horses, for just such a situation. For a retained placenta, a hard bag of hot salt is put under the patient's buttocks, then she must blow through her cupped hands, blow until tired out. The breasts must be kept warm; no water on them, and the best preventative of abscess is a weasel skin to cover them. But if abscesses do occur, remedies used vary from an old man's night cap to autogenous (the patient's own) urine heated and used as wet compresses.

In one such case, three months of such treatment was endured before I came along to incise it and give her sulpha. Jack in the pulpit corms, dried and grated, are considered good for vomiting and gastric upset; in slices, moistened and bound to the sore spot, the patient will be rewarded by a very efficient counter irritant, to the point of blistering.

~

La Jonne, or La Grosse Marie

IT WAS FEBRUARY, a long way below zero, with drifted roads. Seventeen miles to go, but supper was over, and a good team made the going easy. Unknown people, who were in a great hurry. "She has been sick a long time and the baby won't come; it's her eleventh." The trip was easy enough and gave time to watch the stars; think over the day's troubles; rehearse steps to take in view of imagined complications. The old worry, "What shall I do if...?" The first problem was a stable; none nearer than two miles off, but horses have to be stabled. Hermidas had to drive the team off and walk back while I set to work.

It was an arm presentation; the first I had seen. I had rehearsed again and again the steps to take; with no expert help, a low bed, an unknown and very obese patient, mother of ten children, my problems seemed formidable. A turning operation and a breech extraction was, amazingly, easily done. By the time 'Midas got back, had I wished to leave, it was just about time for him to walk the two miles back again for the horses; however, it was better to wait 'til morning.

There were several cases along the way needing attention, and miles were to be saved by doing these before breakfast. Besides, it was many degrees below zero, thirty or thirty-five degrees perhaps. To wait 'til morning seemed best. Then the problem of putting in the time was to be faced. I hadn't my buffalo robes from the sleigh, which had often made me a bed beside the stove in a log hut. In this home, bedding was very short, barely enough for the mother's bed. Besides, the "sage femme" in the district had brought her three-month-old infant with her the afternoon before. It was rolled up in numerous wrappings, and laid crossways at the end of the bench.

There was only the choice between the drafty floor and this same bench. A coon coat helped a bit, but hardly reached from shoulder to ankle. The ankles stuck out, and happened to be just across the finger wide jamb of the outside door. The bench was hard, but not half so hard as the frosty breezes across my ankles. It was not so bad 'til after one a.m., but it was very bad from one o'clock 'til five, when one begins to wake up again. At times the new baby wailed and sneezed promisingly; there was no difficulty breathing. By times, the three-month-old howled industriously, got the nipple, and slept again.

Breakfast came early, as I told 'Midas to have my horses fed early and ready for seven o'clock. It was a long miserable night, but it was the beginning of a long and interesting connection with 'Midas, his wife and family. The next July, when we'd forgotten the thirty-degree temperature of that night, with its cold winds, 'Midas and his wife came to see me.

He, a short tubby little man, sticking his stomach out, hands in his pockets, was looking almost dapper and quite cocky. "Monsieur le docteur, on vous aime beaucoup. You have done a good job in February. Nous en sommes bien contents. But we find that it was too expensive. Fifteen dollars for so little work! La prochaine fois, on n'aurait pas besoin de vous à ce prix! "

I needed the money; I had learned the financial state of 'Midas' family. He was a jealous, lazy, pompous little chap. He attended the storage dams along the creek, trapped muskrats, did really very little to earn a living. She on the other hand, was hard-working and steady, although jealous of her rather worthless little husband. Thus when I insisted on getting my fifteen dollars, she wept a few tears. He raged. Never would I go to his house again; he'd pay like a man; but never would I enter his house again.

With a handful of small bills in my hand, while he angrily folded up his receipt, I turned to his wife Marie, and gave her a two dollar bill. I knew she could use it to good advantage. "Ah, that's good," said 'Midas, "Vous nous faites du bon." "Non, non," said I, "it's for Madame." The fat was in the fire. "If that's the way it is, you can keep her. Elle restera avec toi!" he said as he stormed off out the door, leaving Marie on my hands. Off he went, leaving a very tearful fat woman, mother of eleven children. I urged her to keep the money. "No, no, he'll find out and won't take me home again." She cried; I raged at her, insisting that she keep the miserable two dollars. She left, leaving the offending money lying on my desk. 'Midas had not counted on "la grosse Marie" nor upon a woman's way, and she had her way.

Seven months later she wrote, "Vous tes venu pour mon onzième; venez pour mon douzième." A year later, "You came for my twelfth; would you come for my thirteenth?" And yet again, "You came for my thirteenth; would you come for my fourteenth?" And again and again, up to the eighteenth baby. Never did I miss the call for "la grosse Marie". Never did she give me less than a breech, or a face, or an arm presentation. Never did she allow 'Midas to interfere. She in turn became a "sage femme" and she gave up the polite second person plural and used the familiar second singular, "Tu m'as toujours eu soin, je n'en veux pas d'autre que toi. I don't want anyone else." 'Midas has long gone to his Father's. Madame comes in now and again, after many years, with heart failure, but she always says, "Tu m'as toujours fait du bien."

Marie Ange

MARIE ANGE STOOD ON THE GARDEN path in front of her doorway to greet me as I drove up. Hollyhocks and golden-glow grew against the whitewashed log house behind her; sweet peas and cosmos against the whitewashed palings of the fence about the garden; mignonette, nasturtiums, petunias and larkspur in masses along the path; clumps of hardy phlox, hardy aster and sunflowers in the middle spaces; she stood in a riot of colour and perfume, her face radiant in welcome. Bees were everywhere, crickets sang from across the dry pasture where the mullein grew.

The song of the crosscut saw came from behind the house where 'Mède's old father and his grandson, Philias, cut up the spruce and poplar sticks, peeled in the spring, while Ti Mède piled them into neat rows ready for hauling away. There was no really good crop in this region on which to depend. In wet years, some grain grew; in dry years, little if anything grew. Potatoes often gave a good return; hay was poor and mostly weeds; some years fall wheat gave a crop which, mixed with imported hard wheat at the mill, gave the family flour for the winter. Oats was usually short in the straw and light in the head; many a year, often as not, cut green and used as fodder for the cattle in dry pastures, or for the horse in winter. In a small bottom field near the lake, kept in shape by special manuring, onions, peas, and beans grew well.

The family just made a living from the land, but, were it not for the ten to twelve cords of pulpwood each year, they would have a hard time getting along at all. Pulp gave them the fifty or seventy five dollars cash needed each year to buy tea, salt, and whatever sugar they could not make from their own maple trees in the spring.

It was a lazy hot August afternoon, but there was no laziness where Marie Ange was. "I wanted to speak to you before you came in," she said. "I have Mémère with me, been here three years

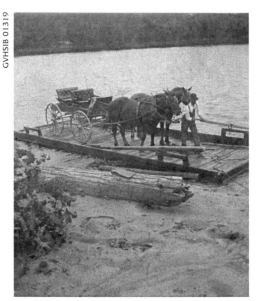

GVHSIB 01319

The too-frequent river crossings.

now; she couldn't look after herself with her sight going so fast. Besides, Pépère helps a lot, works with the boys; it teaches them. I wanted to warn you about her. Fortunately she's a good bit deaf. Don't talk too loud. If she knows you are here we'll have trouble. Le Bon Dieu had pity on me, when he took her mind, he took her ears too."

It was a neat house, whitewashed inside, the Prince of Wales stove shining with polish. The window and door frames were painted a pastel blue, the door panels a dull brown red. Holy pictures hung on the walls. In one corner was the figure of the Virgin and Child I had seen that stormy night by the lake so long ago; in front of Her a lighted candle, and beside, Holy Water. "I have confidence in Her! She has helped me a lot." By the door on one side was the "huche" or breadbox, the yeasty smell of rising bread escaping from around its cover. On the other side of the door stood the water bench with two pails and a drinking mug on the ledge above them; both "huche" and "banc à eau" painted pastel blue to match the window and door frames beside them. In the side wall opened a door to an outer summer kitchen, where a brisk fire kept the kettle boiling. Besides the well-made clean bed, there were on a table, a basin and jug, soap-box, towels, baby clothes, oil and powder, all set out ready. By the basin was half a glass of grains of wheat, to be used as the local belief dictated. About the patient's waist there was a "St. Joseph's belt", a red bias tape of wool, two-thirds of an inch wide, sent from St-Joseph-de-Montreal, to secure a safe delivery.

Every precaution had been taken; it remained only for me to act. Marie Ange's hands were full. "Ma petite cousine had called me to look after her, her fifth in as many years. I could not go to her, so I just brought her here," she explained. "Mémère takes a lot of care. She does not want me to leave her at all. Her sight is gone altogether now. It would not have been so bad if she'd kept her mind. She sits up in bed in the dark over in that room, fingering her beads. She won't let me open the window, even in the hot summer. "I feel a draught, for the love of le Bon Dieu, give me a little water to drink." All her waking hours it's the same, and when I bring a drink, as often as not she flings it at me. She's not really bad of course, she's not herself, she's too much tormented, poor soul."

Meanwhile, the stage was set for the delivery. The afternoon wore on, and by suppertime "la petite cousine" wakened from a deep sleep, to welcome her twenty-minute-old baby. "The poor little girl, she'll have to suffer the same pains as her mother; a little boy gets on better. He can defend himself, and he'll never have the pains his mother has to put up with."

There is something uplifting about washing and dressing a newborn baby; relief and thankfulness that all's well. Even if over ninety percent are born without undue worry, there are still ten percent remaining, enough to try the nerves and prove the mettle.

Bill

Bill was old—his time came that winter. There he sat in his corner, panting, unable to lie down. Driving by in the night, and seeing his light go on, I'd go in and give him a "needle"—rest for a few hours. Bloated, congested, coughing; on and on he went. One night a severe nose bleed kept everyone up; even a square of the priest's robe thrown over his head did not frighten away the blood.

All Bill's best known and most valued remedies had failed. He needed the doctor, and it was forty-two below zero, with drifted roads. I got there and plugged the back of his nose. Mary was grateful—though she was practical too. "He might as well go now and be done with it; he's no good til hisself anyways."

During the many night visits, gradually I got to know Bill very well. At first he was peculiarly stand-offish. After all, he was by way of being a healer himself. There was, on his side, a sort of professional jealousy between us. It was only little by little that I got to know the whole story.

Long ago, Bill, in his youth, had kept the dams at the outlets of half-a-dozen small lakes, reservoirs for spring waters, held there to be let out in summer, as water was needed lower down the valley to keep the saws going. In the early days, the order would come by some passer-by: "Take two stop logs off number five" or "put three logs on number six. We don't need so much water." Bill would do as he was told; as the years went by, Bill gained experience. He seemed to sense when water was enough, or when there was too much. The new manager would hardly need to send his message. Bill could guess, and by the time the message came, the necessary adjustment had already been made—the saws kept going—water was not wasted.

Bill was a valuable man, but in the days of low wages he got little for his pains. It was, after all, a part-time job. Little money, that is, but it was all the same to Bill. He had plenty of time for the life he loved. Muskrat skins, in season, were his for the taking. Muskrat meat took the place of fish on fast days. Now and then a fox, chased by his hounds, would sell for a few dollars. In the fall, a fat bear or two would be his, giving meat for his table, grease for soap, and for sore joints. Beavers, travelling out of nowhere, would settle down and cut off part of his water supply. The level of a dam would fall, or perhaps rise, when it should have been the opposite. Beavers could be helpful, but they seldom chose just the right place or the right time to build dams.

There was continual strife between Bill and the beavers. Many a time he had to destroy their dams to keep his own in order. Great was his satisfaction when the season came round and he could kill off a few for his table, or to get the kidneys, which, soaked in gin, were good for almost all the ills to which mortals were heir.

Long ago the pine trees had been cut for export, long ago the giant cedar had been built into houses and barns and fences by the first comers into the hills. Hardwoods had sprung up, oak and elm, ash and maple, birch and butternut, and made open, shaded areas

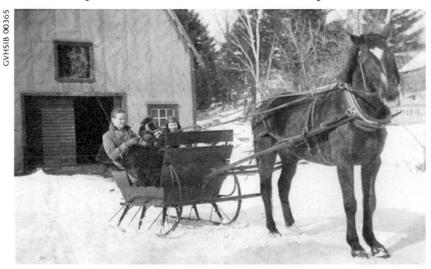

GVHSIB 00365

The Geggie boys—Hans, David and Stuart in their father's cutter, c.1934.

between his lakes, where the shy ginseng liked to grow. Taking short cuts to his dams, under the shade of the hardwoods, he would find the ginseng. Dark-faced Levantine traders, driving queer cartloads of exchange goods, would give good money for ginseng roots. Now and again he might come upon a "forked root", prized by Chinese mothers desiring sturdy sons. At the right season, in the fall, he gathered the corms of Jack-in-the-pulpit; "Indian pipe", he called it. Dried, and ground to powder, he used it for stomach disorders. Dried and sliced thinly, and applied moistened to the skin, a great blister grew, and pleurisy pains vanished. Joe Pye Weed grew about his lakes. When, at its most flourishing, Bill gathered an armful to dry and have on hand in the winter. Joe Pye tea was sovereign for the kidney. Goldthread too, was gathered for ailing stomachs. Maple sugar time came. Bill's sugar and syrup were the best for miles around—boiled in the open pot, with just enough of the tang of wood smoke—there was nothing like it. His cough syrup, Balm of Gilead, and sumac with maple syrup—nothing was so good for winter colds.

His life was full, his satisfaction complete; but Mary came along when he was twenty-eight. Mary was from the village at Puddle Creek Flats; her father "kept hotel". To her, nothing was quite so right as keeping hotel, with its good steady income, the excitement of comings and goings to the shanties. Spring and fall were great times, but all year round there was a coming and a going, forwarding supplies, men coming down on account of illness, and other men going back to replace them. "Have your hotel at the right place, that's all you have to do," Mary told Bill. "There's a good living in it." Reluctantly he agreed.

Married to Mary, she kept her hotel; he his lakes and dams, his bush wanderings and his interests in illnesses and remedies. Mary's hotel prospered; the Lake was the right place, and Mary the right one to run it. She was rough and ready, not without a shady story, a rough word, a frequent pull at the bottle herself. She seemed to know when, of an evening, the right moment had come for "one on the house". When not too many were gathered— it must not cost too much—but when she felt one or other of the company would oblige with a yarn or a song, then she'd call for one on the house. "Shure the gin will get them going." What she really meant was "dang, the gin will keep them coming."

Mary was prosperous in her hotel; Bill was happy with his dams and remedies; together they did very well indeed. Mary expanded her enterprise with cheque changing, and a small grocery and dry goods store adjoining her bar room. While the women picked over her remnants, their men patronised her more convivial bar. Life was easy, interesting and profitable. She was a tyrant, yet her help, fearing her, feared to leave her, and stayed on year after year, grumbling, but they stayed. Nor did the gradual procession of seventeen sons and daughters interrupt her various activities. True, the Good God knew she could not look after so many with her other work.

"Yes, I had me troubles; Bill was never no good to help in the hotel. Him, always away in the bush fixing his old dams—finding his old roots. He never was no good to help out—never one to stop around. The only remedy he had enny good was beaver's kidneys in half a bottle of gin. It's my idee the gin did the trick. 'Twas good for women's troubles and vomiting—in fact it was good where gin was good, that's my belief; his old roots!"

The Fox

I HAD MET MME HUBERT many times. A "sage femme" with lots of confidence in her own powers, rather impatient of the powers of nature, she would walk her patient up and down and round about, hour after hour, until the "moon in her course" had brought the desired delivery. Then she used the burnt rag for the cord; the great scissors to cut the tongue tie; the large teaspoonful of thick castor oil to "cut the phlegm" in the baby's throat; while the mother, with a hard pillow under her buttocks, puffed and blew through her hands to deliver the afterbirth, the cord being tied about the mother's left knee "to prevent the cord going up inside" for "ye'd have nothing to pull on after it was gone." Beaver's kidneys in gin was always ready for after pains. Hand-picked wheat grains waited on the dresser "to settle the childbed, nor must the mother put her hands above her head, nor comb her hair for ten days, nor wash it for six weeks."

Never was an obstetrician more meticulous in her regimen, never was a paediatrician so careful of details. Her patients came through very serious illnesses, all of them with the happiest results. Nor did she let you forget that she'd had sixty-seven babies in her time, never lost one, nor mother either. The rest of us could not say as much. But Madame Hubert was tired.

One hot July day at two-thirty in the morning, the call came; only five miles; a wild colt and a sulky, nothing like it to add spice to life. "Blondie", tied to a phone post, was happy with her nose bag, but she was quite fit to make a get-away, and leave me to get home any way I could. Mme Hubert lay motionless. Was she awake, asleep, conscious, unconscious? No one knew. With a wild shriek in the night, the uncooperative old lady startled her family; they could make nothing of it, nor could I. She lay in bed, wrinkled, thin and sallow; there was always a possibility of brain complications, tumour, meningitis, or mere hysteria, but which?

Day after day she lay there, refusing food, drink, or to talk or pay the least attention to their anxious enquiries.

Many were the questions: Will she get better? How long will she be sick? How long can a person go without food or drink in this hot weather? Many an evasion was needed as I did not know what to say. But at long last, the doctor's best friend, time, came to my aid.

Six weeks had passed, cool fall nights had come. One early morning I went to see Mme. Hubert, and found her as usual, not a change could I see. Why did she last so long without food or liquid? Was she cold, were her feet cold? I felt under the bedclothes; she had her boots and stockings on, laced up over the ankles. "Why did you put her boots on?" I demanded in surprise. "Boots on?" said the daughter, "I didn't put them on." Then Mme. Hubert saw that the game was up, "I was cold—I got up and put them on in the night."

Then the whole story came out. She'd been foxing all these weeks, was tired, wanted a rest. She got up at night and got food and drink, and went to bed again before the family was up in the morning. My words were very much to the point. She never called me again. In fact, never again did she speak to me or look my way if she could help it.

A Day's Work, or Never a Dull Moment

DESPERATE CASES NOWADAYS are given transfusions, even potentially desperate cases have blood standing by for a danger sign. There was a day when this was not so, and a transfusion far into the country was a major undertaking. This patient was bled white from a placenta praevia, a week's steady bleeding, a dead baby. A retained clot as large as the baby itself had brought her too low for transportation to hospital. In any case, there was no money available. I saw her daily, in the hottest part of July, twenty-two miles from my office. She flickered, bloodless, infected, and flat; and she was taking very little food or drink.

At last I phoned a medical friend in Ottawa who readily assembled the syringes needed and agreed to help me. I met him at the station early, prepared to go straight away to see her by daylight, leaving time perhaps to catch a trout when we were through.

As the train stopped in Wakefield, the conductor came running; the trainman had fallen off the steps of the train, and was lying on the right-of-way beside the rails. Away we went and picked the man up, finding that he had a fractured skull, and all the evidence of intracranial haemorrhage. While we were considering what to do next, a severe convulsion shook him. A special train was ordered to take him to hospital, and while we were waiting, we did a spinal tap and got bloody fluid; but he had no more seizures.

All this took time, and it was nearly nine o'clock when we got away on our trip; no fun this time, no trout. As we neared the house, the sky was growing overcast, lightning flashed, and far-off thunder grumbled. Before we could get into the house, about ten o'clock, a full scale thunderstorm had come up, with torrents of rain. We stepped out of the car, and into an ankle-deep stream running round the corner of the house. A whole company of relatives and neighbours had collected to give blood if the correct type could be found. We heard them repeating the "chapelet", a steady drone, "Je vous salu Marie...," rising louder and more hurried as the thunder crashed. The patient, however, was oblivious to all the uproar.

Sampling her blood was soon done; freezing with ethyl chloride to get serum. The first donor rejected, the second rejected, the third, the fourth and the fifth, all rejected. Our supply of ethyl chloride was almost gone; the sixth and seventh rejected.

Finally the eighth cross-matched perfectly. He was a bandit-looking brother-in-law, but his blood suited. We had to run the risk of venereal infection; he denied it, of course. As the storm grumbled, we began our direct transfusion, I drawing the blood from the donor, my friend rapidly injecting it into our recipient. It meant quick work to get ahead of clotting; it required a good supply of warm sterile syringes. Light was essential, and we had

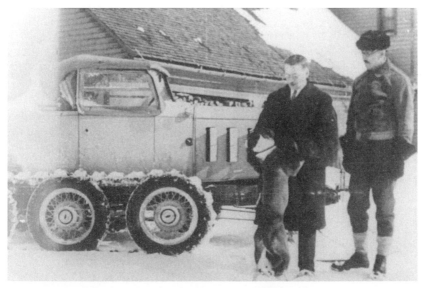

Drs. Harold Geggie and Wallace Troup off on a blood transfusion adventure, c.1930.

133

very little from the oil lamp. At the foot of the wide bed we installed two flashlight holders, flooding each arm with a sometimes adequate light. We worked fast; we had to.

Our light bearers grew faint and shaky, and the batteries began to get low. Still we worked. We lost count of the number of syringes. A syringe blocked and was discarded; a vein was pierced; we had to get another. It seemed an eternity, and all the time the storm retreated in the distance, and the water dripped from the overhanging trees onto the roof and so to the ground. Indeed, it seemed an eternity as one after the other, our supply of syringes blocked and were discarded.

At the end of the time, with very little light, no syringes, a fainting donor, but a somewhat aroused recipient; we had to give up and call it a day. However, there was no reaction.

While we were busy, a neighbour, soaking wet from the storm, brought a message; "Mrs. G. needed me badly, the baby was coming." Needles and syringes were bundled up in a hurry and packed away. Our patient showed some interest in her surroundings, and a little pink in her cheeks; and we were off.

By one a.m. we had the stage set for the arrival of yet another citizen. He did not come 'til an early flush was in the sky, nor did we think of the fun or the trout we had counted upon as we made our way down to the early train.

That all happened in the "lean" part of the 1920s. Last winter, our patient finished her course; third stage syphilis, or general paresis of the insane. Perhaps we saved her life in the 1920s; did we lose it in the 1950s?

Celebration of La-Sainte-Catherine

In France, la Sainte-Catherine, November 22nd, is Old Maid's Day. Horse play of various kinds has been handed down over the years, and no doubt came to Canada with our first settlers. Today the Old Maid angle has been nearly forgotten. "La tire"—pull taffy—has taken her place, and in the country schools at least, teachers with imagination celebrate Sainte-Catherine with taffy boiling on the school stove and the subsequent pulling and eating of the candy.

I was depressed with the grey day, the grey sky, the grey lives around me, and I decided to go home another way, even if it were several miles longer. I would see other farms, other hills, other people, grey also perhaps, with troubles, but at least other troubles. The way led round Stag Creek Lake, on the corduroy road through the swamp, that I had avoided years before going to see Amède. Naturally my thoughts travelled back to that bright day, so full of nature's promise of spring, but the very contrast of that day and this seemed to deepen my mental gloom, and made more oppressive the gloomy barren waste of bush, rock, lake and mountain around me.

All about me was the promise of winter, long and cold and full of anxieties. It spoke of the perpetual daily struggle that can't quite be forgotten, even in summer when the fields are full of ripening grain and the barns are filled with sweet smelling hay; when goldenrod and Indian fireweed fill the ditches and waste spaces with their riches; when flowering milkweed makes the warm air heavy with its sweetness, and grasshoppers of many shapes and varieties bring drowsiness with their endless song. Thus in winter we do think of summer, as in sadness we think of joyous times gone by.

Round the lake at last, the road climbed up a long rocky slope. Frozen or half-melted puddles of mud lay between the boulders on every side, making the car creak and strain every bolt and bar in torment. Up we went, bumping and straining, until all of a sudden, such a clatter set up in the engine, that I knew at once its meaning: lost oil, burnt out bearings. It meant "shank's mare" to telephone for help, and a tow home—twenty-eight miles. Already evening was coming as I started my tramp along the muddy road. Around the horizon a saffron band slowly formed, shining through the greyness of the sky. Far off in the northeast, one mountain top was lit up by a stray beam of rosy sunset. Here and there small half frozen brooklets came hurrying on their murmuring way across the road down to the lake. Mosses and ferns, alone keeping their summer green, were crisp and fresh among the other withered foliage. Lacy hemlocks, cone shaped cedars, towering pines, leafless oak, maple, ash and birch, umbrella shaped elm, all gave interest to the wayside as I tramped along. Evening brought two hungry partridges to the red birch buds, and a silently fluttering woodpecker awoke the echoes with his rat-a-tat-tat in his search of food.

Slowly, breathlessly stopping from time to time, I neared the top of the hill, feet wet and cold, heart pumping away, and breath becoming short. Below in the valley, I could see the welcome sight of a white-washed log house. Even as I looked, a man came out of the bush with a gun on his arm, and a well filled bag over his shoulder. His dog, ever on the alert, seeing me, came barking to the limits of the clearing to investigate, while the man stood in the doorway, looking up at me with kindly interest.

Making my way down towards him, I enquired the distance to the nearest telephone. "Three miles," he answered, "but Monsieur le docteur is not intending to walk all that way? Is it to get help for the car? Then my boy will drive to do the message, while you rest and get warmed up with us. It will be long before the man comes, and you can't do anything until he does. Come in and rest yourself."

As we talked, the door opened, and from it came the familiar figure of Marie Ange. She looked older, true enough, but contented, well and happy. She had recognised me through the window and had come to welcome me. "Come in, come in and rest yourself. The house is not large, but there's room for one more, even if we already have fifteen in it."

"Fifteen, Madame," I exclaimed, "your family must be growing. Who have you taken in this time, and why are you not in your little shop over at the corner?"

"Oh I have not taken in anyone. Telesphore—he's my husband—took me in and all my family. You see, I'm only thirty-five, and life is hard alone. Telesphore too, he was alone since my late husband's sister—his wife, died two years ago. Alone with five children he was. I could not leave him like that; no one to look after his place and his children all winter long when he went to the bush."

As she talked, she made me comfortable by the stove, gave me dry socks, and began to set the table and prepare tea. "I won't get you much, for it's five o'clock now, but at six, people are coming for a dance. It's "la Sainte-Catherine" tonight and tomorrow. The boys and my husband are going to the bush for the winter, and we're having a little dance and making "la tire" to encourage them before they leave—the winter is long you know. Some of them will be home to put in the crop, but the rest will stay for "la dràve", and won't be home 'til the hay is ready to come in."

As she talked, a young girl came from upstairs with a baby in her arms. Smilingly, she invited me to examine her treasure. Marie Josephine, now sixteen, had been married a year to Jean Paul, Telesphore's nineteen year old son. Her baby, already two months old, laughed happily in his mother's arms, as his father prepared to drive to the phone office with my message. The spotless floor, the white walls, the brown ceiling, the purring kettle on the crackling fire, the ticking clock, all showed a prosperity and contentment to be envied, and made a striking contrast to the dullness and gloom of the world outside.

Marie Ange's work never ended. To and fro she went, getting meat to be cooked, looking into the pot stewing on the stove, cutting bread, laying out the table with cake, biscuits, jam and butter and running off milk from the milk can. All the time, her tongue rattled on about the events since last we met.

"Yes, Grandmère, Dieu merci, is gone—found dead one morning last spring. It was funny; she did not want to die, and her so helpless. Seems to me I'd be glad to die if I were like her, yet one likes to live. Grandpère is living. He'll be in soon—he's milking. He advised me to marry Telesphore. He was anxious about Telesphore's children. Then Jean Paul wanted to marry Marie Josephine. She was young of course, but it's just as well to marry when one gets a good man. He is a good chap, steady, and brings home all his pay to his wife. They have three hundred dollars in the bank now. "We had a double wedding last summer, Marie Josephine and I. We fêted the wedding three days, and danced right through 'til morning. When we got through the fête, I hadn't a thing left in the store, so I just locked the door and left it. I brought my furniture and the sheep and even my plants with me, of course. We get along well here together, and now when the men are all going away for the winter, we will have more room and no one will be too busy. Marie Josephine has only her baby to look after, and the little girls will do the housework, while I look after the outside work and do the spinning and weaving. Oh, we'll have a good winter, if no one is sick."

By and by Grandpère and Telesphore came in, one carrying a pail of milk, the other an armful of wood. Lamps were lighted in the gathering darkness, and they and I sat about the fire, talking quietly and smoking, as the women made the final preparations for the party. "Have you looked after your fiddles, you men?"

Marie Ange finally asked. "You know you must be ready, for by the time Jean Paul gets back, he'll be anxious to be 'calling off' the dance. There, take them and get to work, and see if you've forgotten how to play them. You haven't played much since we were married, have you Telesphore? If it weren't for Grandpère helping at it, I do believe you'd forget how to play."

By this time, one by one, the neighbours began to come in, each one with one or two or three babies or small children, dressed layer upon layer, "pour cacher l'air" as they explained. The women laid aside their coats upstairs, and sat rocking the babies and younger children asleep, until one-by-one they dozed off and were taken upstairs, to be put side-by-side on the big double beds to sleep, while their mothers sat gossiping and rocking endlessly. Then the young fellows and their "blondes" strayed in—each couple shaking hands awkwardly, and sheepishly arranging themselves on the benches, holding hands and simpering. Something was needed to liven things up, and that something came in the shape of Jean Paul, master of revels. "The garage man will come," he told me. "My, but the road is rough."

Then we set to ravenously, for the meal was ready. There was a "ragout" of pig's feet with potatoes, partridges boiled whole with cabbages and onions, frozen roast pork seasoned with garlic and sliced thin as shavings, to be eaten with good homemade bread and butter, and there was cream "douce" with scraped maple sugar, sliced raw onions in vinegar, and large winter radishes, big as turnips, to be eaten like apples in the hand; wild blueberry, raspberry and strawberry jams, according to one's fancy, and cranberries too, from the swamps nearby. There were pies of several kinds, and cakes of very doubtful appearance, that went the rounds. And all the time, the kindly jest, the broad joke, the loud laugh, that bespoke the simple lives of these people.

At last supper was cleared away, the table was unceremoniously put outside, chairs were arranged around the walls, and the two fiddlers, sitting in the corner, struck up a lively tune. Five or six bars were played over and over again, as the partners were selected, and took their places for a square dance. When all was ready, the music struck up more lively than before, and the master of ceremonies, Jean Paul, in response to encouragement, began to call out directions, and the dance was on. While certain couples went through special figures, the other dancers jogged 'til their turn came to do a similar figure. Each couple tried, however, to add a special stunt, and some peculiar step, some gesture, some hoot, to liven up the dance.

All the time the jaws kept time with the music, chewing gum gathered by the children from the spruce trees. Old Grandmother Martin, sixty-two she was, danced as ably as the rest, and kept the whole room laughing at her antics. The caller was a hard taskmaster; no mercy had he on the dancers or the fiddlers.

Again and again figures were repeated. Again and again, grand chains were gone through with individual steps, unusual contortions, and couples seized opportunities for individual jogs and violent surgings of partners. Again and again his voice rang out, and the dance went grimly on. At last even he was tired, and the dance came to a sudden stop, and conversation broke out in a quorum. Everyone sought a seat; some found them on the floor, some wandered outside, only to be recalled almost too soon, by Jean Paul announcing another dance.

Finally the event of the evening was announced. Two men carried in from outside a large tub filled with ice from the lake edge, and set it in the centre of the room. Telesphore proceeded to dip from the huge pot standing on the stove, boiling maple syrup candy, "la tire", and to pour it on the ice. All crowded around, dabbing the edge of the candy with a finger or two, to see if it was cool enough to pull. At last it was, and the fun was on. Couples paired off to the tune of much laughter and chatter, and pulled the soft candy 'til it shone golden in the lamplight. Then it was cut up, with a large pair of scissors, into convenient pieces. Some made dolls, or animals, stars or hearts with the pulled candy.

All this took time, and as another dance was called, my garage man honked out on the road for me. An hour later, as I was being towed along the frosty road, the fiddlers were at it again, and strains of "Mademoiselle, voulez-vous dancer," came to me across the fields, to lighten the long road home. Two days later, I chanced to hear that Grandpère, at about midnight, still playing his fiddle, had stopped suddenly for a moment, stared wildly, and crumpled up on his chair—dead. A stroke had come to take Grandpère away from his wood chopping and his hay scything. "C'est la vie," as Marie Ange would say.

Pilgrimage

SHE WAS SITTING IN FRONT OF THE STOVE, the oven door open, her feet resting on a block of wood, trying to get some heat into her emaciated anaemic body. She'd been ill, needing attention, for months. Now nothing but surgery and transfusion would make it possible for her to look after her eight children gathered about the kitchen couch across the room, gathered about Denyse, aged nine, who'd been lying about on account of acute rheumatic fever, St. Vitus dance, a threatened heart.

The children were not upset at seeing the doctor. Long ago they'd got used to "le Père" or "le Vieux", as he was familiarly called. The centre of the group was Louis Marie, aged nine months. Denyse mothered the whole family, but Louis Marie claimed everyone's attention and devotion. A good welcome for each new baby was a matter of course in this house. As the mother continued to lose strength, Denyse, in spite of leg pains and twitching face, took over more and more the supervision of Louis Marie, directing his care in the capable hands of Marthe, aged eight.

Louis Marie was full of little mannerisms, full of posturings and poutings, grins and laughs much beyond his nine months of life and experience. The centre of the group, he continually set everyone off into fits of laughter; clasping his little hands one over the other on his fat tummy; wagging his head, pouting his lips, blowing bubbles, shutting and opening his black eyes, unclasping his hands for a swift slap at one of the group, and clasping them together, again and again; going through his antics, setting us all into kinks of merriment in spite of ourselves. "What funny attitudes to take. I never saw a baby of nine months so wise, so adult. Does he always hold his hands that way?" I asked. "Yes, he does. He's done that for a long time now. He seems to know it amuses the others. I've been too sick and miserable to do much for him for a long time. His father has been away in the bush for months. He always folds his little hands that way, wags his head and laughs. Perhaps it's because I laughed at a priest!"

Later, as I drove her to hospital over the slippery icy roads that bitter cold night, she returned to what was, very evidently, preying on her mind. "Do you think a priest, if he was laughed at, would "mettre un sort"—cast a spell on Louis Marie? It's not natural for a nine-month-old to behave like that; it could be a spell, couldn't it?"

"How did you come to laugh at a priest, Madame? Did he get angry at you? I don't believe a priest would, even if he could, put a spell on any woman's baby. In any case he is a very happy jolly wee lad. I wouldn't, if I were you, think of it again. But how did you come to laugh at a priest?"

Then, as though to unburden her conscience before the uncertainties of surgery, the whole story came out. She was the penitent—I the priest. "You see, I was two months gone with Louis Marie. I was always an excitable creature, and I suppose I should have stayed at home when I was like that, but Albert was drinking a lot; all that family does. I had to do something about it; with my eighth coming I had to stop him somehow. Believe me, with seven needing food and clothing, and another coming, it's disheartening when your husband drinks. He's good to me and makes good wages, but all his family drinks too much. The damned drink; I had to do something, hadn't I?

"A pilgrimage was to start at five in the morning from Ottawa for Cap-de-la-Madeleine. Sophie, my neighbour, was going, trying to obtain a favour from Notre Dame. She wouldn't tell me what it was, but I thought it must be the favour of a son. She was getting old—forty two. There was not much time left if she was to have a boy, after nine girls. I was discouraged. I had to eat early, as soon as I woke, or be upset all day. To go on the pilgrimage meant that I would have to start out fasting, and not eat 'til after Mass and Communion at Cap-de-la-Madeleine. I didn't know if I could do it, but I took no lunch with me, not even my cigarettes and matches, so I would not be tempted. I wanted to make a good pilgrimage. I'd never been on the train before.

"Just imagine, twenty-seven, and never been away from home. You see I was married at seventeen and my baby came soon after, so I never had time to get away. I was a bit afraid to go by the train; but the more sacrifice I made, the more likely Notre Dame would help me obtain the favour for Albert. It did help him too. He drinks less now, but I want him to go on a pilgrimage himself next summer; that would cure him. Do you think I'll be well enough to go with him, or will I be dragging around waiting for the next baby by the summer? I hope I'm better by then and able to go with him, but I don't want to lose this baby either. Sophie and I started at four o'clock. Albert left early with a load of wood, and dropped us at the station in Ottawa in plenty of time, but I was hungry, and I wanted my cigarettes. However, the station was full of pilgrims.

"Soon we were allotted to a compartment. I don't know how many compartments full there were, but each one was in charge of a priest to lead the devotions all the way down. We said twenty four Rosaries before we reached the Cap!"

"Did you eat nothing all the way down, nor smoke?" I asked.

"No indeed, the priest gave us no time for that. If we weren't saying the Rosary, he was reading the lives of the Saints, or telling the story of Notre Dame du Cap and the building of Her Church long ago. After a while—I suppose I was tired and weak, but I began to laugh and could not stop. I tried to say the responses more attentively, say them more loudly or faster than the rest, but in spite of everything, I'd start to laugh and have to hide my face in my handkerchief. The priest was so funny. He had a funny round face; he was fat and short and bald, except for a small tuft of hair in front, hanging part way down his forehead. He had small, very dark, bright eyes in his fat face, and his nose was flat and spread all over his face. Then he had a habit of shaking and wagging his funny head from side to side as he led the prayers. Besides, he clasped one hand over the other across his fat stomach; then he'd unclasp them again and again, without end. It seemed as each prayer ended he'd unclasp them, and clasp them again as the next prayer began. I could not help laughing in spite of the prayers, but I did manage to hide most of it, on the way down. Coming home, after High Mass and Communion and a good meal, I made up my mind to choose some other compartment. I hoped to have another priest for the home journey. This, to my sorrow, I found to be impossible; each of us belonged to his own compartment. There were no more prayers on the way home—we were all tired; nothing to take up my attention.

"Every time the priest looked my way I would burst out laughing in spite of myself. I was ashamed, but I could not stop it. That little bunch of hair on his bald head; his little black eyes; his wagging head, his flat nose, his fat cheeks, and his hands. It was all too much for me. I couldn't help it, I had to laugh, and he caught me at it. Is it any wonder my baby is such a queer little chap? The priest must have wished it on me. Later in the summer, my neighbour on the other side, seeing what favours Sophie and I had obtained from Notre Dame—Sophie was already expecting the hoped for boy, and Albert had stopped drinking—she decided to go too, and see if Notre Dame had a favour for her. When her compartment leader asked her where she came from, and found it was my Parish, he immediately enquired about the woman who laughed so much.

"He remembered me. True, he asked how I was, hoped I was well, and had obtained Notre Dame's favour. He was kindly, but he remembered me; me, one of hundreds he had met. I'm sure he cast a spell on Louis Marie. They are so much alike. He might have been the boy's father. Maybe some day Louis Marie will direct a pilgrimage to Notre Dame. Maybe it is a good spell the priest cast on him."

We were at the hospital door by then. There were other things to think about.

~

On Being Fed in the Country

In the name of the best restaurants, and of good company, and of turbot pie, alas! In our world, one goes in daily expectancy of eating to live—one is, so one must eat! Red-letter days come at irregular intervals, and, as one sits around the table, with the family of eight or ten, and with food enough for fifteen or twenty, one thinks of epicureans, and has no reason to be jealous. "Sit in and make out your supper," is the order of the day, and when one has gained that comfortable lazy feeling which comes of hard work, and long fasts, well broken, one's host remarks: "Have some more pie; there's nothing much on the table, but try and make out your supper." This comes at the end of pea soup, venison, with potatoes and tomatoes and parsnips, pickles and relishes of five varieties, salmon loaf, bread, white and brown, with butter, cakes and cookies and buns, iced and marbled sweets such as the King never tasted, pies of three kinds, cream, apple and raisin, with whipped cream; as well as honey of the best, maple syrup, last year's blackberry crop, tea with cream. A red letter day indeed, when one feels lazy, and the evenly heated, large clean kitchen, honest and welcoming faces, the sweet influence of children, make the journey home seem light and easy, and not long and dreary as anticipated.

Red letter days come at intervals, when one wonders just how much food it will require to sustain one's activities; to do the day's tasks, to keep one's mind master of one's body, to make the body obey the mind—when one works against the inevitable oncoming of meal time—when one thinks of excuses that will satisfy one's too hospitable hosts—when one sizes up the preparation of the meal with swift glances, and surveys with mingled hopes and dismay the contents of the pot, and the burden of the table. Gradually, as the minutes pass, one's supply of ready made excuses runs down; eagerly new ones, less elaborate, are made. Anxiously one scans the household faces to discover how far credulity has been strained—how much they have been offended. "This is my fast day," or "I never eat between meals," or "I've had my dinner already." No excuses will do.

With ceremony, the white, more or less white cloth, often a sheet, is spread; after the green tea dust has been boiling madly for half an hour on the heat warped stove, after the eggs have been fried and fried, and solidified like well-used rubber soles, fried in grease that has done nothing all its life but fry and fry; after the very salty, very thick, slabs of pork have been par-boiled in water of uncertain cleanliness, and fried until they are stringy and tough as leather; after the butcher knife has been wiped on a dirty greasy dish towel, and the bread has been cut against the dirty dress of the hostess, or her equally unclean daughter.

Alas, one sits, excuses gone, hunger and exhaustion rampant, nature calling loud for fuel to accomplish the daily tasks. The tea is poured, scalding and black, bitter, with brown sugar to sweeten the tannic acid, but no milk. One takes a spoon, dirty, and with a gulp, the scalding tea is stirred, while one wonders at what temperature and for how long, the associated millions of germs will succumb. A dish piled with slabs of pork, like chips of last year's chopping, smothered in eggs that resist assault, is passed around the table. Each one removes his knife from his mouth, or from his dish, or wherever it may happen to be, and helps himself to as much as his stomach can hold, and then some more. Your turn comes, and with another gulp, the far side of the dish, as yet untouched, is tried, in the fond illusion of securing a first-hand supply. Then comes the pot or bowl of soggy, often cold, potatoes, and the same brotherly method of service is enacted. Following this, one must sample the butter and bread. One begins to consider just how this particular supply of butter came to taste just as it does; one wonders how in the name of Creation it is so spicy. In dismay, one picks away at egg and pork and potato, one tries and tries again to wash something down with the tea, and keep a straight face at the same time.

All around the table goes on the most wonderful knife play, making the lightning journey from plate to mouth and back again, in perfect safety. Forks are used only as a lion would use his paws to hold his victim, while the knife replaces his teeth in doing business with the meat. With increasing signs of gloom and dismay on one's face, and equally evident signs of satisfaction and repletion on that of the host, the meal drags out its inevitable and too long delayed end. Again, one's host exclaims: "There's nothing much on the table, but try and make out your dinner." It's true, there's nothing much left; nor is there in a cornfield when locusts have passed. Once again, having failed miserably, one wonders how to stick it out 'til the accomplished task permits a hasty and welcome retreat. One dines at the best restaurants, but one is fed in our world.

Forgotten

"WHY DID YOU LEAVE IRELAND?" I asked. "Because the poor man had no chanst there," Paddy replied. And in that short sentence was compressed all the bitterness, all the feeling, which his one hundred and six years had been too short to smother. There he sat, propped in his Morris chair, a faded artificial-fur cap, like a mutton pie, on his head, his few bits of dirty, white, straggling hair only half concealed. His deathly grey, shrunken face was animated only by his fadeless blue eyes, in which still gleamed that droll cunning so often seen in the Irish, at intervals his pale, drooling lips gave issue to short, meaningless, explosive utterances.

At times the whole man took on a death-like immobility, and apparent insensibility, as though he were already looking beyond, and exploring the possibilities of the next world, before entirely letting go of this one. Suddenly, his old claw-like hands would begin to grope about aimlessly, and with the aid of one of his daughters, Bertha, his pipe would be found and lit. With the old glint of humour animating his features again, he would announce, "I'se bin smokin' for nigh on a hunnerd years." Watching him there, hunched up on his low chair, dressed in indescribably patched and ragged clothing, with an old Irish shawl pinned about his shoulders, I pictured to myself his coming to this world of ours, aged twenty-two. Was it possible that this pathetic, almost repulsive, old fellow was ever twenty-two? Was it possible that he ever found his desire answered by the love of a mate? Was it possible that ever in the past this poor old wreck looked with pride and love and awe, mixed with fear, upon his first born?

Was it possible that in this old shrunken breast, ambitions for his nine children ever stirred? Was it possible that in the long past his life was such as to earn the love and devotion and care which I saw lavished upon him? Was it possible that one hundred and six years ago, a mother, in an Irish home, looked with tearful, although forgiving eyes, upon this newborn babe, now grown so old, so distorted, so almost inhuman? One must have a large sympathy to recognise the realities of such a life, to admit the unity of human experience, to acknowledge the brotherhood of man.

Like an old Scottish lady, who in her sad, deserted, very old age, used to exclaim aimlessly, "The Lord be angered wi' me. The Lord ha' forgot me; He winna let me die." So it is with old Paddy, the Lord ha' forgot him, He winna let him die."

Neighbourliness

I was heading to a new patient, forty-five miles from home; over a new road, up beyond Balm of Gilead, over the divide looking down into the far-off valley of the Picanoc River. A new world: time was to be saved by taking a guide, evening was not far off.

Gérard was the only pick-up not busy, not busy because of his precarious heart condition, a heart that was to get slowly worse, and by spring, end his time of waiting—a young acute rheumatic, with leaky valves, waiting for a final acute attack that the colds of winter would almost surely bring. A guide, but certainly not a helper in time of trouble on an unknown road.

Ernie Starr was bleeding from his stomach ulcer; time was important. We talked little, Gérard and I, as we threaded our way from the village along the winding bush road, past a shack where hardwood logs were piled up on a rollway, past cords of pulpwood, and piles of hard cordwood for city furnaces and fireplaces. All were waiting for the eager trucks, nosing their way through the bush. "Virez à droite," remarked Gérard, as we came round a large rock and saw a mere track through the hardwood bush, not a very likely road to take! But my guide was a native, and I had to trust him.

Yard by yard, as we went, the road became worse and worse, swamp on either side, across unbridged rivulets, and over slow-moving swamp water. There was no chance to turn; what a place to live! Through another and another soft spot, until, with a sickening, sucking sensation, we settled down in the king of all bush mud puddles, there to rest, both axles in the almost bottomless swamp.

Evening was already coming; nothing to do but walk on and see if someone could help us out. Gérard could not be asked to push or handle the car, or even to put blocks under the jacked-up wheels. His long lean face, almost girl-like good looks, straggling fair hair, slightly bluish lips, and broad clubbed fingers, showed conclusively, his inability. Walk on, I must, perhaps see my patient, and so lose less time. Some way we'd get out, some time!

Giving Gérard my lunch, and telling him to stay quietly in the car, I set out over the sodden bush road: whippoorwills began their noisy evening contest, far off, near at hand.

Cicadas ground out their discordant rattle, shadows lengthened as I hurried along, momentarily expecting to see the Starr house around the next bend, see my patient, get help, and get on the way home. Mile after mile, and I still kept on, no house in sight. Yet it was a distinct roadway, for I could feel it with my feet, even if I could not always see more than the strip of sky between the tops of the overhanging trees. Stars began to glimmer, no use to go back, it was too far. Perhaps around the next bend waited my patient. Tired, hungry, stumbling in the growing darkness, I kept on.

Gradually a light seemed to glimmer through the tree trunks ahead. Then the sound of wood chopping gave encouragement to my wanderings. Not to take the chopper by surprise, to announce my coming, I called again and again; but the chopping went on. The motions of the man, for I could see him now quite plainly, made the lantern light flick on and off as though he was signalling to someone far up on the back mountain.

All around was dark as I advanced towards the light, calling out vainly to attract his attention. As I got close up, I saw my man, rough, dirty, and unkempt; dressed in incredibly patched coat and pants, hair long, tousled and filthy, ugly, but not in a nasty way. I felt half afraid to approach, nevertheless I had to get help, I had to see my patient, I had to go on. I almost had to touch him before he could see me! Stopping, his axe in mid air, a hobgoblin look about him in the pitch black open doorway of his woodshed, lighted up by a smoky lantern; Stephen looked at me. "Oh! Who are you! Where do you come from?" Perhaps he thought me an apparition, as I was half inclined to think him. No doubt, in the fitful light, with the dark bush behind me, I, too, was apparition enough. Explanations offered were little understood, Stephen added deafness to the rest of his uncouthness. At last he was voluble enough.

The Starrs? I was long past it. This was the last house on the road. Beyond was the Picanoc valley. There was nothing after that. Yes he'd help me. The Starrs were good neighbours. He'd help, but first he must have his supper! "Come in and wait while I eat. Have you eaten?" One glance at the room he took me into decided me. I could not eat there.

A box of rosy red apples stood on a chair, all else was piled up with the accumulation of years, newspapers, boxes, old harness, empty bottles of patent medicine, ointment boxes, everything grimed over with the dirt, not of days, but certainly of years. In the corner, a bed of sorts, a "lounge", he no doubt would call it, was piled up untidily with quilts. Close by was a wide, spreading Prince of Wales stove.

From a grimy cupboard he took a piece of a loaf of bread wrapped in incredibly dirty newspaper, a piece of cheese, also in dirty newspaper, a sticky bottle of molasses with dead flies still sticking to its sides. Sitting down on a box by the table, he set to. "Sit in and make out your supper", was his invitation, but although hunger gnawed at me, and although I knew that I'd need fuel for the long walk back to the car, I could not face it. I lied cheerfully, or as cheerfully as possible; I'd had my supper as I walked along, I'd eaten my lunch! "Well have some apples then, I've just picked them and they're good." Good they were, and many of them helped to tide me over; somehow the dirt of wind and weather seemed less than the human dirt of everything else.

"Well, we'll be going," said Stephen when finally the last crust of bread, the last morsel of cheese, and a good part of the molasses had vanished, washed down by the cold tea left in the pot from dinner time. "We'll be going, but first I must get my axe, you carry the lantern," he ordered. "Why" I shouted? "Well we might meet a bear as we go along. I seen one a few days ago and they are nasty at this time of year, eating up for the winter." Stephen seemed wound

GVHSIB 00362

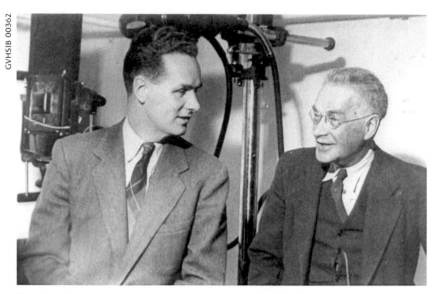

Dr. Hans Geggie with his father Dr. Harold Geggie, at the opening of the Gatineau Memorial Hospital.

up on that trip back to the car; nor could I add anything to the conversation because of his deafness. The long shadows cast by my swinging lantern on the dark tree masses were spooky as my companion told one long-winded story after another; wood lore, habits of porcupines, of bears, of foxes and wolves, of caribou and deer and moose; about neighbours and their families and his brother up in the Timmins mining area, his plans for fixing his house, and fishing trips.

By the time we reached the car I knew all about Stephen, his way of living, his philosophy, his acute bush sense, his neighbourliness, his independence and reliability. With all the rough exterior, here, beyond civilization, was a heart of gold, neighbourliness, kindness, and independent ruggedness. But as we reached my mired car we heard voices! I had left Gérard in the car eating my lunch, with whom was he talking?

Then lights shone through the trees and the bulky sides of a team of horses and many men came into view. "Get the team around here! No use to pull it ahead. There is no chance to turn there. We'll draw her back. Hitch on here." As we came into the circle of light, Hiram Peck came up to me: "You come with me. Starr's is not far from here, through the bush straight across here. The rest will get your car out. Your patient may need you bad." Another of the Peck family took charge of getting my car out of the mud; Hiram, swinging Stephen's lantern, started off through the bush, giving me a hard time to keep up with him.

Through a fringe of bush, over fallen logs, around great boulders, down a twenty-foot ridge of rocks, across a creek and over a field of grain, where the stooks stood like ghosts in the pale light of a rising crescent moon, through two barbed wire fences, and a garden of cabbages. At last Starr's house came into view, set on a little high ground in the midst of an old beaver meadow.

As I went over Ernie Starr's long story; through the thin partition I could hear Hiram Peck explaining to Mrs. Starr how I'd taken the wrong turn, and how the neighbourhood had roused to help me. "We saw him pass our house, and your dogs did not bark as they always do when a car comes along. We knew he had taken the wrong turn; young Gérard must have made a mistake. So we all came along to help him out. As the doctor was so long coming back, Bert Mulligan thought that Ernie must be very sick and that help might be needed. As he passed the turn off, he noticed that the car tracks took the wrong turn, and concluded that the doctor had gone on to Stephen Early's, and that he must now be stuck in the bog; so he went back to get his team and a few other people. They'll be having the car out to the road now, and someone will drive it here to get him very soon."

It was long past midnight when I, at last, got home; but I'd met new people, new problems, and I'd seen how a hardy people make life easier for each other. I'd met new friends.

Prescription for Twelve GPs

TAKE ONE GRADUATE NURSE, of good and sufficient experience. No objection if she's good to look at.

—Take one trained attendant, a good cook and a good housekeeper.

—Take one social worker, male or female, expert in rural life, trained in city work.

—Take one good midwife, of infinite patience and endurance, if possible a mother. Rub these four together, and set away to mellow.

—Then take one well-trained physician, one interested in infant feeding and paediatrics, in acute infections and fevers, knowing smallpox, well versed in typhoid fever, interested also in T.B., cancer, cardiology, allergy, and having an aptitude with degenerative and chronic cases and old people.

—Also take you one surgeon, long on diagnosis, especially abdominal and gynaecological, short on using the knife, but resolute, sure, and swift when he does. Interested he must be in orthopaedics; and he must know the possibilities of neurology, gastroenterology, urology, major and minor traumatic surgery and so on. He must be a practitioner of what I shall call "destructive dentistry"; in other words, he must be able to yank out a tooth, or a dozen of them, with or without local or general anaesthetic.

—Take, too, a very good obstetrician, one having the good qualities of a midwife, one not too surgically minded, one able to row a river, climb a mountain, and do his stuff solo, with a fainting husband, a coal oil lantern, and a mattress on the floor. One of these two must be a good anaesthetist, knowing the smell of ether, but well versed in the use, perhaps the abuse, of chloroform. He must know the use of sedatives, and be able to use modern intravenous Nembutal, Pentothal, and Nitrous

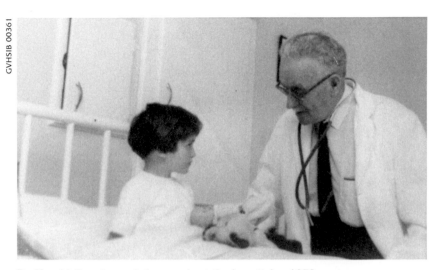

Dr. Harold Geggie on daily rounds at the hospital, c.1952.

Oxide. He need know only enough about the modern explosive anaesthetics to leave them alone.

—Take you one good eye, ear, nose and throat man, one who sees further than the tonsils and their removal, one who knows that mastoids can still be infected in spite of antibiotics.

—These three must be thoroughly versed and interested in pharmacy. There is no better way to save money for you and your patient than to know as much as you can about the drugs you use, or the drugs you make your patients buy. Then shall you rub together these three professionals, and also lay away to mellow.

—Take also one good sanitary engineer, one well versed in drainage systems, sewage, water and milk, food and air supply.

—To him add a psychologist, one interested in psychiatry, but one who has not gone whoring too long after the modern concept of sparing the rod to avoid child inhibitions! I believe in inhibitions—else how could we get along with each other? Also take a good lawyer, one with a sense of humour, able to make wills, knowing the transfer of property, the rights of women, the protection of children, and the control of men.

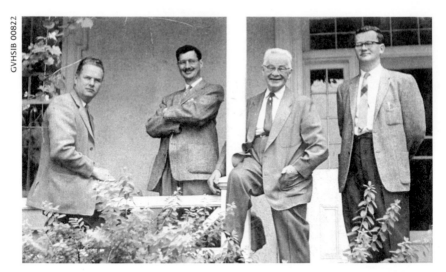

Doctors Hans, David, Harold and Stuart Geggie at the Gatineau Memorial Hospital. 1956.

—Lastly, take one good priest, of any convenient sect, of liberal theology and wide sympathy, and perhaps humour; one able to baptize, give ghostly counsel, and to bury if need be.

—Rub these four together, and add to the former mass, and stir together lightly. It would be a mistake to mix it up too thoroughly to a uniform consistency, for no one wants all GPs to be of a pattern. Thus in one would the surgeon predominate; in another, the midwife obstetrician; in yet another, the family, municipal and social counsellor.

—These, spread freely across the landscape, at twenty to twenty-five-mile intervals; with or without hospitals or other help—except it be a good wife! Thus will you bring modern medicine to the people. Thus will you make specialists and hospitals worthwhile.

The Last Mile —
Editor's Postscript

D R. GEGGIE'S LIFELONG GOAL WAS TO ESTABLISH *good health care in the community, and with this in view he spoke to numerous organisations, pleading his case for health education for mothers and their children, better public health measures for food handlers, milk and water supplies, and, of course, sewage disposal. In the 1930s, he spoke to a Women's Institute group, advocating rural hospitals and visiting nurse programs, as is now known and taken for granted over much of Canada.*

At the end of hostilities in 1945, with his eldest son returning from overseas to work with him in Wakefield, and his two other sons studying medicine at McGill, Dr. Geggie threw his energies into the promotion of a community hospital as a fitting memorial to those who died in war, as well as those who served.

On March 2nd, 1952, the Gatineau Memorial Hospital was opened, with twenty-two beds, and six bassinettes for newborns. It was and is, in every way, a community effort. Before opening day, donations of bedding, home-canned food, vegetables, and labour, were generously supplied by people from miles around, and on that great day a long line of supporters waited in cold March temperatures, to see their hospital.

Since then, the Gatineau Memorial Hospital has continued to grow, and add an ever-wider range of medical services. In spite of two attempts by provincial authorities to change its status and function in the community, it is stronger than ever. At a public meeting held in the Roman Catholic Church in Ste-Cécile-de-Masham, where bureaucrats and politicians were present, some two thousand people attended from a radius of thirty miles—almost one-third of its population base, speaking French or English, the desires of the

GVHSIB 00328

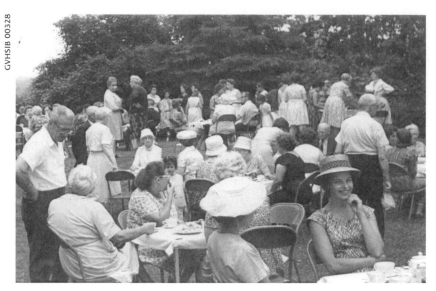

Annual Garden Party at the Gatineau Memorial Hospital, c.1958.

population were eloquently expressed and debated; the people had spoken.

Harold Geggie's contribution did not stop with health care. He served as Mayor of the Municipality of Wakefield Village for two terms, and was instrumental in the planning and the construction of a new school in Wakefield in 1941, while serving as Chair of the School Board for many years.

Dr. Harold Geggie died in 1966, at the age of almost eighty years, and after more than fifty years of practising in the Gatineau Hills.

In his Will he established the Dr. Hans Stevenson fund with a donation of $10,000.00, to be used for scholarships for local students who aspire to go into the health field; medicine, nursing, or medical technology. Thus Dr. Harold paid tribute to the "Old Doctor", as well as promoting good health care in the community. This fund has been used over the past forty years by students in dietetics, medicine, nursing, and X-ray, amongst other fields.

In 1996 the Gatineau Memorial Hospital relocated to a newly constructed building on Burnside Road in Wakefield. It continues to serve as a "teaching hospital," allowing medical students and resident doctors from McGill University to gain experience for extended periods of time.

A name change was made to Wakefield Memorial Hospital to avoid confusion with the Gatineau Hospital in the nearby city of that name. In 2006, an integrated health-care system was introduced, with the Masham, Chelsea, Val-des-Monts and Cantley CLSCs, the La Pêche Nursing Home and the Wakefield Memorial Hospital amalgamated into one health-care delivery organisation, called the Centre de santé et de services sociaux des Collines *(CSSSC).*

A Hospital Foundation has long been established as the fund-raising arm of initially the hospital; and now, known as Des Collines Health Foundation, it continues to support the hospital, the CLSCs and the Nursing Home.

This system serves the wider community which had been the "stomping ground" of Dr. Harold Geggie for fifty years. As his determined effort was for the betterment of health care in the entire community, it is rewarding that the system appears to have come full circle to now offer a service of which he could only dream.

A bronze bust, executed by noted sculptor and Gatineau summer-resident, Harold Pfieffer, has been moved from its location at the original Gatineau Memorial Hospital, and now stands in front of the new hospital on Burnside Road.

In MacLaren Cemetery in Wakefield, a granite boulder marks the graves of Harold and his wife Ella Stevenson Geggie.

It bears a quote from a patient: "He came when we needed him," and under Ella Stevenson's name, a quote from her husband of over fifty years: "Without her t'were not possible."

Acknowledgments

I WOULD LIKE TO EXPRESS my gratitude to John Hardie, who has revived "The Extra Mile" in his remarkable and sensitive presentation of "Dr. Harold" a clever portrayal of the man who devoted his career to the community; and I am also grateful to the Wakefield Players for their contributions to these performances. My thanks go to Zoé Lindsay who efficiently brought this into print once more and with whom it has been a pleasure to work. Adrienne Herron generously devoted much time in supplying pictures from the Gatineau Valley Historical Society's image bank, and Anita Rutledge greatly assisted with her editing. I thank the *Ministère de la culture et des communications du Québec* and the Gatineau Valley Historical Society for financial assistance in the production of this publication. As well, I am grateful to my many friends and members of my family for their encouragement and help.

Norma Geggie, 2007

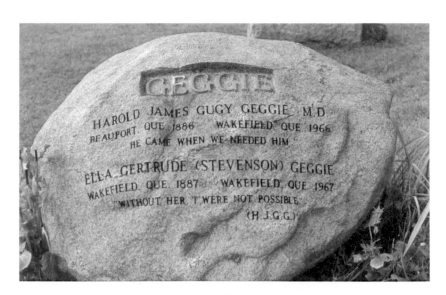